About *Still Bigger Than Pink - Alive and Thriving:*

Still Bigger Than Pink is a beautifully written book. It touches your heart and soul, and could only be authored by an angel like Lori Lober. Out of the pain and the suffering she went through comes this beautiful light that shines on us all. This book is a must read for all women in America. I loved it.

Dr. Tony O'Donnell, ND.
ABC, NBC, CNN News Reporter, 2000
Leukemia and Lymphoma Society Man of the Year, 2001

What people are saying about Lori Lober's first book:

Bigger Than Pink, The Book I Could Not Find When I Was Diagnosed With Stage IV Cancer.

Anyone who has ever met Lori Lober has had their life enriched by her passion and dedication to life. I have treated hundreds of cancer patients and survivors and have helped them answer the hanging question: ' *Ok, I survived, now what?!'* In all of my years as a doctor of chiropractic and a wellness minded healer, I have never met a person more willing to be a coach and a friend for the people who call upon her experience. Lori has an amazing passion for helping others and is willing to share her personal trials so that someone who hears the dreaded words 'you have cancer,' will have an idea of what is in store for them. Bigger Than Pink is a great read for anyone who is feeling that scare in the pit of his/her stomach that seems to happen with life changing events. Read it and then follow the action steps that are listed in each chapter. Cancer can be beaten, my friends, and on̶̶ ̶̶ ̶̶lopt a wellness philosophy answering ̶̶ ̶̶ ̶̶hat it never comes back again, and so that you can live the high quality, fulfilling life that you deserve.

Dr. Bruce Rippee, D.C., C.C.W.P.

I became a cancer survivor in July of 2008. I knew very little about it and feared for my life. I worried about my family and loved ones too. I began to realize this was bigger than me and I needed help lots and lots of help. I strive to be a strong independent woman, so I had to swallow a little pride to ask for help, in all aspects.

Amazingly people came out of the wood work! People I never knew, complete strangers ready to help. At the beginning of my chemotherapy I crossed paths with Lori Lober. I then began to understand that I am now on the journey of my life.

I read her book during treatment, "Bigger Than Pink". I was at my lowest point with chemo. I had no energy level and severe bone pain. There were times that it felt like it would never go away. So I would read some chapters over and over for reassurance. Lori gave me strength in knowledge, and survivorship. I'm learning to filter out the toxins in my life, and striving to live healthy and whole. Before I was diagnosed, I was just living, just cruising along in life. Now, I am really alive. I have been touched by cancer.

Jennifer Heath, Stage IIIb Breast Cancer Survivor

Once I picked up BIGGER THAN PINK I couldn't put it down! Lori's honest and straight forward approach to her battle with cancer was truly inspiring. I applaud her for talking about how she was able to view physical changes from cancer and put her happiness first. The resolve that she had to beat her disease gave me ideas on how to fight my own cancer and the strength to live a healthy lifestyle. I couldn't wait to set up acupuncture treatments.

Thank you for writing such a helpful book. It has helped my healing in many ways.

Jeri J. Wood
Breast Cancer Survivor

Dear Reader,

   <u>Bigger than Pink</u> is just that. *Bigger than cancer.* In 2003 I received the diagnosis of early stages of hepatitis C. I contracted the disease some 20 years earlier as a surgical nurse. I have and continue to use the book as a road map in my wellness journey. The strategic life style changes and complementary modalities have made my treatment easier and my outlook on this life changing experience a positive one, most of the time. Let's keep it real. It's really a hard thing to do, day to day's end.
   I have been very blessed to be with Lori in her wellness journey. I knew her b.c. {before cancer}, and have been amazed and in awe of how the words "you have cancer" have changed her life and so many others'.
   Now I am on my own journey into wellness with Lori by my side. It was so much simpler just being a wellness buddy. Keeping myself front and center on the path has been made easier by my forever friend's steps leading the way. For this I am forever grateful.

Laura Myer

   Four words changed my life forever: "You have breast cancer". The Cancer had never shown up on any of my regular mammograms, and it was only after having an elective surgery that they realized I was already Stage III. Within 10 days I had three surgeries to remove fourteen of my lymph nodes and both of my breasts, which was my choice. "Emotional" doesn't even begin to describe how I felt. But if those four words changed my life, then <u>Bigger Than Pink</u> completely changed my attitude towards the disease.

The book was nothing short of inspiring – I knew after reading it that if I was going to beat this thing (and I'm a fighter, so that was never even a question), I needed to change my attitude. It is so important to be informed when you're battling Cancer, and while doctors are obviously valuable sources of information, Survivors have been at the front lines, and they will help you fight and hold your hand every step of the way. Lori Lober was my hand holder. She helped me adapt a treatment program that included nutritional, holistic, and traditional approaches. On August 20, 2008, my 62nd birthday, the results from my first PET scan revealed that I am currently cancer-free. I owe so much to Lori and her wonderful book. It has made all the difference.

Kathy Koehler
Stage III Breast Cancer Survivor

Dear Lori,

What a blessing you are, & how grateful all of us at Holy Spirit are that you would share your story with our Women of Spirit group. I hope you felt the spiritual hug, love, & blessings of our group for you and your beloved last night. I just want you to know that Colby's smile, love, and inspiration continue to live through you! God bless you all forevermore!

Anette Growney

Dear Lori~

I am so glad I finally had the opportunity to meet you last night at Genentech's "HER STORY" program! You did a fabulous job! It was very moving.

Thanks again for writing such a great book. As you know when you are first diagnosed with a life threatening illness, you want to read everything about the disease. I finally stopped reading the technical books about cancer and picked up your book instead.

I especially loved the fact that you talked about complementary therapies. I truly think there is a connection with our mind, body and soul. Thank you again for writing a book that made a huge difference on me and my cancer journey.

Michele Murphy, CEO & Founder, www.pinklemonadegal.com

What energy! What strength! What spirit! I was instantly in awe over her story the first time I met Lori Lober. I knew God had a reason for me meeting this awesome woman. After reading her book I knew I needed her to share her story with my students. I wanted my students to feel the empowerment and strength of someone who had weathered so much and was not just surviving but **THRIVING**!

Lori's story, her book is not just for those with cancer, it is for everyone that wants to feel empowered, everyone that has lost hope in their lives, everyone that wants to be the best they can be. Thanks Lori for your willingness to share your incredible journey!!

God Bless!

Judy Frueh WHNP, BC

STILL BIGGER THAN PINK

Alive and Thriving!

BY

LORI C. LOBER, CSP, MIRM
FOUNDER, TOUCHED BY CANCER FOUNDATION

WITH TERESA M. KELLY

COVER DESIGN BY: MICHELLE RIERSON

authorHOUSE®

AuthorHouse™
1663 Liberty Drive
Bloomington, IN 47403
www.authorhouse.com
Phone: 1-800-839-8640

DISCLAIMER - The information in this book is provided for educational and informational purposes only. We are not attempting to prescribe, treat, or recommend and in no way is the information contained in this book intended to be a substitute for a health care provider's consultation. If you are ill please consult your own physician or appropriate health care provider.

First published by AuthorHouse 5/15/2009

ISBN: 978-1-4389-7016-5 (sc)
ISBN: 978-1-4389-7017-2 (hc)

Library of Congress Control Number: 2009904443

Printed in the United States of America
Bloomington, Indiana

This book is printed on acid-free paper.

Portions of this book were previously published in Bigger Than Pink, The Book I Could Not Find When Diagnosed With Stage IV Cancer by Lori C. Lober, CSP, MIRM with Lara Moritz, first published by Author House 10/07/05.

IN LOVING MEMORY OF MY SWEET ANGEL IN HEAVEN
AND ONLY CHILD,
COLBY JAMES McLAIN AND ALL OF MY FAMILY AND
FRIENDS
WHO HAVE LOST THEIR BATTLE TO CANCER.

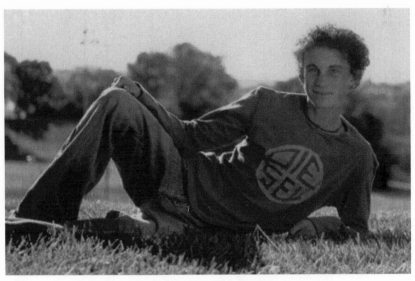

Colby Photo by Tracy Routh Photography

For My Brother, Lance Cory Wittmeyer
January, 1965-May, 2000
You Are My Angel!

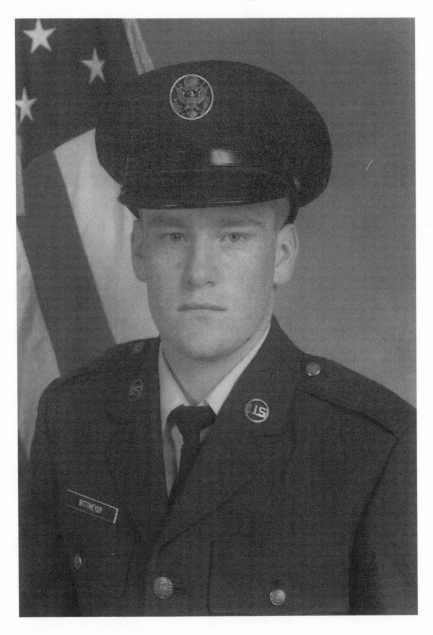

The power of story never ceases to amaze me.
My heartfelt gratitude for all of you, whose stories touch
and enrich my life,

and,

With deepest appreciation to Lara Moritz, Len Lehman,
Sandra Duncan, Denise Evans, Teresa Kelly and
Laura Myer
for helping me bring my story to life!

Thank you John Lober for being by my side – through the good
times and the bad.
I look forward to many more wonderful moments with you in
the years to come!
I love you with all of my heart!
XOXO

Table of Contents

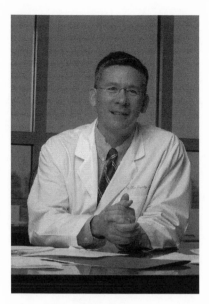

Dr. Lyerly

Foreword

By H. Kim Lyerly, MD
Director, Duke Comprehensive Cancer Center

I had been searching for Lori Lober for some time. Lori had participated in a clinical trial for advanced stage breast cancer patients at the Duke Comprehensive Cancer Center in 2002. My colleague, Dr. Michael Morse, and I were following up on all of the patients who participated in the trial to ask about their lives after 5 years. We had contacted all of the women in the trial, but could not reach Lori. Finally, I personally called Lori's current phone number. When a woman answered the phone, I hesitated. After all, when I met Lori, she had stage IV metastatic breast cancer. Based on the statistics, she was not supposed to be alive. I asked the woman if I could speak with Lori Lober. "I am Lori Lober," she said.

On the phone with Lori, we talked for a while. She had been on an extended trip and had just returned when we spoke. I became reacquainted with this inspirational woman as she told me details about her life since her participation in the clinical trial, all of which is chronicled in this book. She began the story with her diagnosis – and her difficulty in being diagnosed -- and ended with her life today as a cancer survivor and patient advocate. Lori's story is one of hope and determination, and this book tells it well.

Lori took control of her destiny immediately after her diagnosis. She researched clinical trials, investigated complimentary and alternative medicines, and sought treatment at comprehensive cancer centers. She has become an outspoken advocate of clinical trials. As a breast cancer surgeon and director of the Duke Comprehensive Cancer Center, I share Lori's support for clinical trials.

In my view, clinical trials are one of the fastest and safest ways to find treatments that work against cancer. Most new drugs for cancer will take 12-15 years and millions of dollars to test for safety and efficacy before they can become available to the public. Clinical trials enable patients to have access to cutting edge treatments and new therapies.

All of the women who participated on the clinical trial with Lori were advanced stage breast cancer patients, and all are alive and well today.

Lori uses her book to educate others about complimentary and alternative medicines and about terms such as National Cancer Institute designated "Comprehensive Cancer Centers." There are only about 40 such centers in the United States. As defined by the National Cancer Institute, Comprehensive Cancer Centers must conduct and integrate research activities across laboratory, clinical and population-based research.

"Still Bigger Than Pink" is a great resource for others who have cancer or who have a loved one who is battling this disease. Lori takes you -- with heartbreaking honesty -- through all of the trials and tribulations of her journey with cancer. Because of her candidness, we as readers of this book, live the highs and lows with her and learn from them. I am in awe of patients like Lori who are given this devastating diagnosis but refuse to give up. More than that, Lori relives this difficult time in her life and shares it for the greater good. This book gives others hope. As a physician and researcher, her story inspires me to do more, to keep working, to never give up on patients, and to never allow my patients to give up on themselves.

My best wishes to Lori and to all of those courageous patients who have or continue to battle cancer.

Sincerely,

H. Kim Lyerly, MD

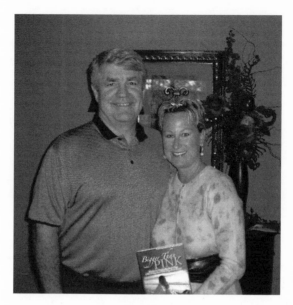

Dr. Geier

Original Foreword

"Bigger Than Pink"

By Larry J. Geier, MD
Medical Oncologist, Kansas City, MO

I first met Lori Lober in 2003 at a symposium focusing on the prevention and early detection of breast cancer. She was one of many women there that day, many of whom were breast cancer survivors. But for some reason she stood out among the crowd, and her questions and comments after my presentation were right on the money and greatly appreciated. We both came away from that encounter with the feeling that, "Gee, he/she really gets what this is all about." I knew that she and others had created the "Touched By Cancer Foundation" in Kansas City to help current and future cancer patients in a variety of ways, and I sensed in her a level of energy and commitment that I couldn't help but admire. However,

I really had no idea until I read this book just how admirable a woman she truly is.

On the surface, the book is an accounting of her trials and tribulations in fighting Stage IV breast cancer, including the things that went wrong, and the things that went right. Since her cancer was invisible to the mammogram, there was an unfortunate delay in her diagnosis. She had difficulty identifying a team of doctors with whom she could communicate in the way that she wanted, and that she could trust would be providing aggressive state-of-the-art care. Ultimately she achieved an amazing result, in that she is cancer-free now, five years out from her diagnosis. (As of this printing in 2009, Lori remains "no evidence of disease" now, nine years since her original diagnosis.) That accomplishment is remarkable in itself, no matter what the path to get there.

However, this book is much more than a mere chronicle. It is a window into the person Lori really is, a woman with great spirit, and a remarkable will to survive. She didn't just beat the odds to get where she is today; she refused to accept those odds, and was determined to do whatever it took to give herself the best chance to beat the cancer. This included not only the best and most aggressive therapy that traditional or "Western" medicine had to offer, but also a combination of complementary types of treatment not routinely used in cancer care. Among these were such things as acupuncture, reflexology, herbal medicine, colonic cleansings, and therapeutic touch and massage.

Most of us American-trained physicians know little or nothing about these alternative treatment modalities, and tend to have a certain level of mistrust of them because they don't seem sufficiently "scientific" for our liking. That usually means that we haven't yet figured out a way to measure them scientifically, and thereby "prove" a cause and effect relationship between the treatment and a beneficial outcome. In my opinion, we even tend to be somewhat arrogant in our view, daring to call what we do with surgery and medicines "traditional," while designating treatments that have been used successfully for centuries as "alternative." Some of us are perhaps more open-minded, and prefer to "integrate" the best of both worlds whenever possible, for the maximum benefit of the patient. I certainly don't claim to adequately understand how some of these modalities work, but I have indeed seen them work in many patients....helping to control pain, to relieve stress, to improve nutritional state, to maintain energy, and to apparently bolster the immune system. I honestly don't know if they help to fight the cancer directly in some way we can't yet define, but I know all too well the limitations of chemotherapy, radiation, and surgery, and frankly, I can use all the help I can get. I do prefer to know when my patients are considering such therapies so that I can help to guide them the best I can, but I know I still have much to learn. To that end, this book has been quite helpful, and I have learned much from Lori's descriptions of the various treatments she included in her program, why she chose them, and the benefits she received. It might be that a different combination would be effective in different patients, but these are surely a good place to start.

Presumably you are reading this book because either you or someone you care about is battling cancer. If so, I believe you will find it to be both instructional and inspirational, a rare combination. Lori alludes to Lance Armstrong and how she found his book to be inspirational to her, but I believe if their positions were reversed, he would say the same thing about her writings. Lori once asked me if I thought she was truly a "cancer survivor" since she had Stage IV disease and is still taking active therapy. No one can say for sure whether she is truly "cured" or is living in harmony with her disease, but it is certainly true that for some people cancer is best viewed as a chronic illness requiring chronic management. Either way, in my view Lori is the absolute personification of the phrase "cancer survivor". I find her spirit and determination, her ability to integrate the best of traditional and alternative medicine, tailored to her own needs, and her willingness to give to others without hesitation, all to be remarkable, admirable, and truly inspiring.

Larry J. Geier, MD

Medical Oncologist

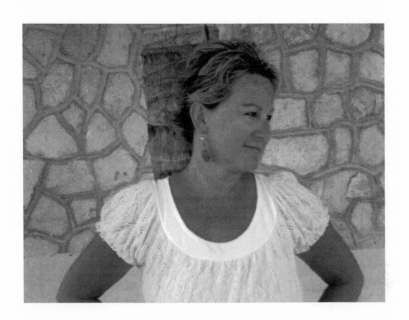

A Note From the Author

Cancer is a battle you have to fight within yourself. In order to become whole and well, you have to find what you need from inside. Even family and friends, as much as they want you to get well, can't do it for you. You have to find the strength deep inside yourself, or you're just not going to beat it otherwise.

I'm not a hypochondriac, but in the 1990s, I knew something was wrong with my body. I was told, however, after my third mammogram that there was no sign of cancer; come back when you're 40. I was 38 then, and had been chasing this for two years.

I can't stress enough how important it is to keep on searching for answers. You cannot be 100 percent certain that something is not cancer until it is biopsied. My doctors missed the diagnosis three times and three different mammograms missed it as well. I could have been really ticked, but in the long run, I wanted to stay focused and put my energy into getting well. When you're told you have a two to three percent chance of being alive in five years, you've got to bring out the big guns, and fight like hell.

After my positive biopsy, I went to a comprehensive cancer center, and was diagnosed with Stage IV breast cancer with metastasis to my liver. That was one of the worst days of my life. My doctor told me the traditional therapy that was FDA approved at that time, offered me little or no hope. He said, however, that he had a spot left in a clinical trial and I would be perfect for it. I said yes immediately – and I didn't even know anything about clinical trials. The way he explained it, it was a no-brainer. I believe I was lead to that trial – I don't think there are any accidents when it comes to something like this.

The trial was designed specifically for women diagnosed at Stage IV and HER2+ node-positive. In the trial, I took a pre-adjuvant Taxotere/Herceptin chemotherapy cocktail for six months before my double-mastectomy surgery. I had no reconstruction. They wanted to make sure the metastasis was shrinking before they even worried about the breast tumor – and it did.

After my mastectomy, I had to continue to do chemotherapy because I still had a cluster of cancer cells in a lymph node they had removed during surgery. I had officially finished the clinical trial and then my oncologist prescribed the traditional FDA-approved Adriamycin, Cytoxin, 5-FU regime. After that I would do four rounds of Navelbene.

That November, in the time between surgery and chemotherapy, I decided to escape the holiday stress and spend Thanksgiving in Cabo San Lucas with my son Colby and my mother. What better place than the ocean to heal and spend quality time with my dear Colby? We rode tandem bicycles, played in the pool, and walked along the pristine beach. On November 21st, we celebrated his birthday. He shared with me often that it was a wonderful getaway that he would never forget. Those heartfelt memories continue to be a source of strength for me to this day.

After the trial and the traditional therapy were completed, I wanted to know what else was out there. The experts always recommend over-treating cancer the first time, so I went on the Internet and found another clinical trial on my own – one that involved a cancer vaccine. I took the information to my oncologist;

he took it from there and contacted the lead investigator at DUKE Comprehensive Cancer Center. After further testing, they accepted me. In my mind, this was dotting the i's and crossing the t's.

From the very beginning in addition to my "Western" medical treatments, I added complementary modalities. I found a nutritionist at a holistic center in Kansas City right after my diagnosis, and she explained to me how to eat properly and begin to empower my immune system.

I also pursued the benefits of therapeutic massage, reflexology, acupuncture and colonics. For me, embracing the complementary modalities reassured me that I was doing everything in my power to build and then to keep my immune system whole and well.

My family and friends have been my cheerleading team through it all, and my son, Colby, was my number one cheerleader. I think about how positive he was at the time of my diagnosis and throughout my treatments. He would say to me over and over that he knew I could beat this disease.

I continued to embrace my healthy lifestyle, passing each screening and test, remaining "no evidence of disease." I was happy living life from a new perspective and helping others to have hope in the face of a cancer diagnosis. Nothing had prepared me for the next turn in my journey. Late in November of 2005, I lost my son and only child Colby in an early morning auto accident. With the outpouring of love and support from my husband John, my best friend Laura and all of my amazing friends (you know who you are), I was able to keep my head above water. My deepest gratitude goes out to those who gave me the strength and courage to move through the grief and overwhelming sorrow that felt as if it would engulf me forever.

Searching for comfort and strength, I returned to the ocean for healing, this time by the shores of Malibu. My heart opened to the healing and newness offered by the rhythms of the ocean. I felt the waves of grace and rebirth washing over me. Reading my own words in *Chapter 1: The Power That Lies Within* helped me get through this heart-wrenching time. It helped me to renew my dedication to being well and being present for my husband and dear friends in my life. I continue to embrace the healing power of the ocean and treasure the memory of my son's playful abandon. Loving and living in these oceans and life experiences that connect us all, I treasure every memory of my sweet Colby. These will never be taken away!

While in Malibu I saw my Tibetan Monk, Dr. Yeshi Dhondon. I had been seeing him regularly for five years then! He assured me that while from an Eastern medicine point of view, my liver and gall bladder were compromised, (most likely from the stress and pain of losing Colby, my sweet Angel), that in his opinion I remained "no evidence of disease". He gave me a new prescription for Tibetan herbs that he wholeheartedly believed would alleviate the A-Typical migraines plaguing me as of late. (Western medicine also confirmed my current diagnosis of "no evidence of disease" within weeks upon my arrival back to KC!)

Today I remain "No Evidence of Disease." Since I participated in my first trial – nine years ago – the FDA has approved the pre-operative chemotherapy. In 2007, I was invited back for a follow up of the vaccination program at DUKE; the success of it had been phenomenal, and it has since moved on to another phase of clinical trials. I can't imagine not participating in these clinical trials when I did. I believe it is one of the reasons I am still here, alive and well!

I have never had anything given to me my entire life. You've got to make things happen yourself, and I think a cancer journey is the same thing. Throughout my journey I've learned that you've got to believe that you're going to beat it with every ounce of your being! If you believe it and see it you can beat it!

Journey Well,

Lori C. Lober

Introduction

My journey is "Still Bigger Than Pink" and it is about being "Alive and Thriving!"

Who am I and why I am I writing *Still Bigger Than Pink*? The answer to the first part of this question is fairly straightforward. My name is Lori Lober, I live in Kansas City, Missouri, and I partner with my husband John in the new home-building industry. I am a wife, a mother, and a stage IV cancer survivor. The answer to the latter part of this question is a bit more complex. In April 2000 when I was diagnosed with metastatic breast cancer, I searched everywhere for hope and help – for a better understanding of my illness and ways in which I could combat it. I read everything I could get my hands on. There seemed to be no shortage of books about cancer and terminal cancer patients.

I encountered stories of triumph and inspiration. Richard Bloch's story was a great one. The fact that he was from my hometown helped somewhat, and I know he helped many cancer patients. However, my greatest source of inspiration came in the spring of 2002 when I read Lance Armstrong's book, "It's Not About the Bike" (if you have not read it, I highly recommend it, regardless of whether or not you are fighting cancer). Reading about Lance and his struggles and ultimate success battling cancer, gave me hope (although I did not have it when I truly

1

needed it – if only I had his book sooner!). Lance Armstrong, in my mind, is "super-human", and by learning of his strengths, extraordinary gifts, and successes, I found my own strength. He has served as my hero and inspiration throughout my cancer journey.

Unfortunately, these stories were more the exception than the rule. Much of the information I found seemed to be either out-dated or "far-out". Many of us have seen and heard of the crazy ways some believe cancer can be cured. I even read about how drinking my own urine would cure me! I continued searching. I read numerous stories, books, and articles written by cancer patients – many of whom ultimately died. This naturally depressed me, leaving me with more questions than answers. Witnessing my younger brother's battle with cancer had taught me that my own life now depended on being proactive. It was time to take matters into my own hands.

After my diagnosis, I began pre-operative chemotherapy ("chemo") immediately. Once I became comfortable with the multi-disciplinary team of physicians at M.D. Anderson Cancer Center (MDACC) in Houston, Texas, I felt totally confident that my recommended course of treatment would offer the best chance for long term survival. First, five months of pre-operative chemo was necessary to shrink the tumors as much as possible, since the cancer had already spread throughout my lymphatic system and I also had two tumors in my liver. Three months later, the liver tumors were shrinking. In September 2000, I underwent what was then an experimental surgery called radio-frequency ablation. The physicians explained that rather than performing surgery, ultrasound-guided radiated therapy to the tumor would offer me greater hope. The team at MDACC believed it was a success, but only time would tell. (Over eight years later, I now hear what was then an experimental procedure is referred to as a mainstream treatment option). After a three-week "vacation" from chemo, I underwent another cycle just prior to undergoing a double-mastectomy with no reconstruction in November 2000.

A positive prognosis is more likely when the cancer is confined to the breast(s). After cancer has spread (metastasized) throughout the lymphatic system and forms distant tumors in other critical parts of the body (e.g. the liver, brain, lungs or bones) the prognosis becomes far more complicated. I mention this because throughout my journey, especially in the beginning, many reassured me, "you'll be ok". They believed this because it seemed as though everyone knew someone who had breast cancer five, ten or even twenty years ago and "they're still doing great!" It was only after I would ask these same people, if in fact, the cancer had metastasized, most had to confess they were uncertain.

While I was confident about the treatment I was receiving at MDACC, I continued to search for what seemed to be good ideas or additional modalities I could incorporate with my prescribed "Western" medicine treatment. Beginning in April 2000, beating cancer became my fulltime job. What else at this point could be more deserving of my time and energy? My chemotherapy treatments continued, and I devoted one full day each week to that. Throughout my journey (and believe me, it's not over) I have incorporated many complementary treatments. Based on my research and reading, I began to receive therapeutic massage every Tuesday, acupuncture on Monday, Wednesday and Friday, and reflexology on Thursday. I also traveled to M.D. Anderson Cancer Center monthly as well. This was necessary since I was participating in a clinical trial. As you can see, I was very busy. I believe this was ultimately very beneficial to me, since it left precious little time to feel sorry for myself.

On January 1, 2001 (01-01-01 --- a sign?), feeling poorly from the chemo, John, Colby and I were watching television together. I stumbled across "DATELINE", the NBC television show. The entire hour was dedicated to the story of Dr. Yeshi Dhonden, a Tibetan monk who specializes in treating metastatic breast cancer. He had also been the personal physician to the Dalai Lama for over twenty years. Dr. Dhonden comes to the United States once a year from Dharamsala, India. I felt I had to see him and I did. I've been a regular patient of his since October 2001. I have taken Tibetan herbs recommended by Dr. Dhonden, three times each day since then. As a matter of fact, it was Dr. Dhonden, my Eastern medicine physician, who first declared there was no cancer in my body during that first visit! (His pronouncement was confirmed by my "Western" medicine physicians shortly thereafter). Of course, we discussed diet, exercise, herbal supplementation and many other things. I would need to continue to do "everything right" for a very, very long time in order to keep the cancer from "wanting" to invade my body ever again.

I continued chemotherapy as well. My acupuncturist told me he was going to prescribe SHOU WU WAN, a Chinese herb, to make my hair start growing back. I thought we were experiencing a breakdown in communication. I said, "No, you don't understand. I am going to continue receiving chemotherapy for a long, long time". He replied, "No, I do understand. In spite of the continual chemo, I am going to make your hair start to come back." I bought the herb, I took it and my hair began to come back. (It was great having my own hair when my husband John and I renewed our marriage vows at the height of my chemotherapy treatments on our five year anniversary!) I still think my oncologist was a little freaked out each month I saw him at MDACC— the stage IV bald lady from Kansas City had hair!

I turned forty years old October 31, 2003. In 2000, my odds of seeing my fortieth birthday were very slim (2-3% chance of survival, at best). So, it truly was a milestone for me, my family, and friends! I'll always remember my "spa trip" to celebrate with some of my closest friends, and my surprise birthday party with many dear friends present! In 2005 I wrote *Bigger Than Pink, the Book I Could not Find When Diagnosed with Stage IV Cancer*. I was telling my story so much it made sense to chronicle my journey in a way that it could spread the message of hope and empowerment to many others touched by cancer.

I am now celebrating 2009 having just been declared NED (no evidence of disease) by my oncologist once again! The last nine years of my life have been spent fighting cancer. However, my fight goes on. My wellness journey evolves as I listen to my body's signals for what feels right to keep me healthy. I continue to receive a therapeutic antibody (Herceptin) on a regular basis. (It does not kill fast-growing cells like hair). In total, I received Taxotere/Herceptin in combination for seven months, Adriamyacin, Cytoxin, 5-FU and Navelbene for four months each. I have undergone six surgical procedures (two eye surgeries were needed because of increased tearing from all the chemo) and an unbelievable amount of tests. Today, physicians' appointments, screenings and a wide variety of wellness appointments are a continuing part of my journey.

This brings us back to why I have updated and revised my first book. I wanted to share the ways in which my journey has evolved. Woven through the original *Bigger Than Pink* is new information about what I have found to keep myself healthy and thriving. I simply want to help as many people whose lives have been affected by cancer as I possibly can. I made a promise to God to help others when I first realized the gravity of my diagnosis. Before, during and after each periodic test I undergo to determine whether or not the cancer has returned, I have reaffirmed that promise.

I'm updating my story with the hope that it will make someone else's journey easier. I spend many hours every week telling my story to patients, their friends and loved ones. I have spent countless hours at luncheons, dinners, and other functions/fund-raisers, conversing with fellow cancer patients. I have found that they are all hungry for information, guidance and a real-life success story. Perhaps I can be that success story and convince other cancer patients to seek out all their options. Perhaps they will join me and become success stories as well!

I am not a medical doctor. I have received no formal training of any kind relating to medicine or health. I am, however, a fighter. I'm an ordinary person who has made beating cancer my long-term goal and thus far I'm alive and well. Is it the chemotherapy? Is the Herceptin I continue to receive keeping the HER-2 NEU (the oncogene that fed my very aggressive tumor) in check? Did the 100+ herbs, vitamins and supplements I took for the first seven years play a role? Has drinking green (or red or white) tea regularly and eating a "properly combined diet" been a factor? Is the IsAgenix cell cleansing and nutritional system helping my immune system daily? Has my unwavering faith in God and my continual meditation played a role? My physicians cannot tell me for certain. What I do know is that I will give you an honest account of my journey and if this little book can help even one person beat cancer, one of my dreams will have been fulfilled and I'll be tickled pink!

Chapter 1

The Power that Lies Within

"I saw myself as whole and well on the other side of my treatments."

In April 2000 when I was diagnosed with stage IV breast cancer, I went through a period of shock that produced many mixed thoughts and emotions. Most of my thoughts caused me to worry, and most of my worries caused me to fear. It is important to understand that these feelings are normal for a newly-diagnosed cancer patient. At first such feelings may seem negative, but they can be channeled into positive feelings and a positive attitude. If you are about to become a "world champ fighter", jumping in the ring with the fiercest of opponents (cancer!), then a positive outlook is the best of allies.

I began to view my worries and fears as the fuel that would ignite determination, intuition, work ethic, and conviction. I worried about what would happen to my family and friends if I was no longer there for them. I also worried about how and where I would die and in what manner I would be put to rest. I actually began to plan my funeral.

I visited a psychologist, and she explained that it was very healthy and natural for me to be experiencing these thoughts and feelings under the circumstances. At first, I had a difficult time understanding how this could be healthy. Then I realized I was simply afraid of dying. I began facing my fear of death. It was human nature for me to worry that I was going to die, but recognizing and confronting my fear helped me to arrive at a greater and more beneficial understanding: *"everyone dies at some point, but there isn't anyone on this earth that can predict exactly how long I have to live."* Cancer can certainly be life-threatening, and it does not necessarily have to be life-ending. I understood, embraced, and believed in the possibility that I might survive. I turned worry and fear into hope and belief, which then enabled me to develop a positive outlook. I was then able to channel hopelessness into constructive thoughts that would help me find and focus on a path to recovery. Positive thinking will provide the foundation for inspiration and guidance, to always stay the course and to never give up. Understand that negative and even heart-breaking news can fuel you throughout your struggle to beat cancer. I realized that even the most helpless situation can be reversed and transformed into power. Hopelessness can be countered by conviction, control and the realizations that the mind is extremely powerful and sometimes it is possible to achieve the seemingly unimaginable.

"Cancer wants to kill me". I had to put this thought out of my mind. If I allowed it to take over my emotions and attitudes, then it could weaken my resolve, and be a drain on the "fuel reserves" I was building. Cancer is an obstacle that often appears overwhelming and impossible to overcome, but I firmly believed that I was strong enough to do so. I saw myself as whole and well on the other side of my treatments. I visualized my physician saying, appointment after appointment, "You have no sign of cancer in your body."

Hopelessness does not exist in the mind of a positive thinker, so I got rid of it. Instead, I came to realize how in control of my life I could be, regardless of the presence of cancer in my body. The daily reality of living with and fighting cancer offered little hope, but taking control and becoming determined to live and live well, filled my heart with hope. I persistently searched my soul for every ounce of belief that I could muster. Every minute, every hour and every day became opportunities to live, learn, and grow as a wife, mother, sister, daughter, friend and cancer patient. I learned that when we can clear our Qi —our emotional body — of counter-productive and life-distorting matter and emotions, healing is accelerated and life becomes more purposeful, joyful, and fulfilling.

When I heard the words, "you have cancer", my life seemed to crumble before me. I was thirty-four years old when I first found the suspicious lump in my breast. Following a mammogram, I was told not to worry, that it was only fibrocystic disease, which approximately 75% of women are diagnosed with at some point. Needless to say, I was relieved to hear that it was something that was supposedly very common and treatable. But for the next two years, the lump grew larger, and the pain surrounding it, although not always present, became more intense. Deep inside, I knew something was wrong. I didn't obsess about it, but I did think about it often despite several more trips to the doctor, mammograms, and breast exams, the results of which were all negative.

In spite of that nagging feeling I had that something was very wrong, my eventual diagnosis (metastatic breast cancer that had progressed to the most severe stage), was still an incredible shock to me. Cancer had spread throughout my lymphatic system and to my liver. My husband John and I could not believe what we were hearing. The results of a mammogram just one week prior to the diagnosis, indicated "no sign of cancer – please return for another mammogram at age forty" (that would be in another three years). I was angry, for I could not understand how both mammograms and physicians' breast exams could not produce a timely and correct diagnosis. I had been misdiagnosed for two years during which time the cancer had spread and progressed to the most terminal and severe stage of metastasis. At this stage of diagnosis, I was given an estimated eighteen months to live and a two to three percent survival rate for five years.

My misdiagnosis and statistically poor chance of survival left me with little hope and waning confidence in conventional medicine alone. I read every book I could possibly find on the topic, and most left me sad and listless. Things were not turning out the way they were supposed to. However, herein is a perfect illustration of the power of positive thinking! I was angry with the doctors. I was angry that three mammograms failed to detect the cancer, when, in fact, my breast tumor was almost the size of an egg. I nearly allowed my anger to negatively affect my opinions about doctors and conventional Western medicine in general. This most definitely would have been the wrong path to take. In my opinion, and I believe most would agree, conventional Western medicine is essential in the treatment and survival of cancer. Having negative thoughts and beliefs during my search for the best conventional treatment could influence my decision-making and lead to an overall negative result. So I chose to redirect my inner energies away from anger and disbelief, and toward a useful, productive and (and ultimately rewarding) action-oriented state of mind. Consequently, I considered the end of my two-year period of misdiagnosis as a call to action. It was time for me to take control of my treatment plan, and I now felt that my survival was entirely up to me. There are many physicians who treat cancer daily, but naturally, there is no one as focused on my survival than I. At this point I knew that I had to find a Comprehensive Cancer Center and a treatment team that would be working for me and not on me. I knew that I needed to get the ball rolling since according to statistics I had relatively little time.

Affirmations and Angels. I will admit, it was extremely challenging for me to draw anything positive from the unpromising statistics of my diagnosis. Physicians clearly conveyed the message that I was most likely going to die sooner rather than later. Therefore, I decided to acknowledge the statistics as a reminder of the significance that I must play in my survival. I jumped into the ring and started fighting. I became highly competitive in proving the statistics wrong. I was not a statistic and I refused to become one!

Since then I have also learned there are cancer survivors who are alive and well today - every type of cancer - every stage of cancer!

I used affirmations in order to continually empower myself and remain motivated. I would say them aloud and to myself throughout each day, especially when I felt that my positive thinking was being challenged. (Although I now have no evidence of disease in my body, I continue to do this daily). This is another method I used to remain focused on the path to recovery.

One must control one's mind, then the mind can control the body — this was my mantra. I thought, "Lori, if you are constantly thinking negative thoughts you will have a negative attitude. You are a human being with a powerful mind, body, and spirit. You are capable of overcoming anything!" I would assert that "my body is whole and well" or "my body is happy, healthy and whole" every morning when I would wake up and every night when I went to bed. I also made these assertions whenever I had a few free moments to meditate — waiting at various appointments, while undergoing scans and x-rays — every extra little bit of time I could find. Even when I visited the bathroom I would envision the cancer being flushed down the toilet!

I gave continual thanks daily for all that I had to feel happy about: my marriage, my wonderful son, a great family and friends! Now my gratitude is also for simpler pleasures, like being able to witness the sunshine glisten off the snow on a winter's morning, as if God Himself was telling me "everything is fine." Perhaps we are too often distracted by the rigors of our daily lives to notice when God is trying to remind us that He is there, He is watching and we are important. In graciousness, we let God know that we believe and in our belief we find purpose. My world before cancer had never been this beautiful. It is amazing how my senses came alive after being diagnosed with a life-threatening illness! I remember when I took such great pride in being a career woman, firmly on the path to bigger and better things in the new home-building business, and the great importance I placed on those goals — that all seems so distant now.

I have a strong belief in the presence of angels among us here on Earth. The image of an angel with wings hovering above those in need comforts me. In the depths of my battle against cancer, I came to believe that God would place a white feather from the wings of an angel for me to see, so I would continue to believe in the purposeful beauty of my life.

God has filled my soul with hope in the representation of a white feather many times. This first occurred while on a vacation in Jamaica following three months of exhausting chemotherapy in the summer of 2002. While in Jamaica, I read Lance Armstrong's book, **"It's Not About the Bike"** which brought me great hope for, and reaffirmed my belief in my survival. (I later flew back home to the U.S. thinking of the story of Lance's triumph over cancer).

At one point during the trip, a friend and I stopped to pose for a photo in a garden overlooking the beautiful Caribbean Ocean. I felt so connected to Lance's book that I clutched it and held it close to me while the photo was taken. Afterwards, we looked down and saw a white feather lying between us at our feet. We glanced up and noticed that there was not a single bird in the sky. Somehow, this seemingly insignificant event touched me with an overwhelming sense of meaning. It gave me a feeling of strength which brought belief, the recognition of a friend who supports my belief, and a God who believes in me. This was reason enough for me to believe in myself. I believe that if you keep a watchful eye, then you will find moments such as these everyday. Pay attention to everything that brings you joy and then give thanks. If you find reasons to be thankful for life, you will find strength to face the adversity that challenges you. Find reasons to live. Recognize the blessings that have been bestowed upon you and use these gifts as reminders of why you want to live.

The struggle to beat cancer was an emotional roller coaster for me. I could not avoid having negative emotions, but I did refuse to allow them to consume me. I conquered them with my desire to live. Every feeling, emotion and experience in life happens for a reason. The future is determined by how one chooses to deal with them. I used affirmations; I prayed, gave thanks and I converted every experience into positive energy. I was going to do whatever it would take to survive.

From Resolve to Action. In the summer of 2002, I was finally sure of myself. I had received a bundle of awful news, and I managed to overcome my negativity and create positive energy. I had developed conviction and a resolve to win the fight, which was a result of knowledge and understanding. With strong conviction and belief, I was able to be courageous and take action – nothing heroic mind you, but acting upon my conviction without fear of failure. I channeled my actions in a positive way to underscore and support my beliefs.

In addition to positive thinking, I found that an action-oriented attitude and focus is required in the fight against cancer. Survival must now be my number one priority. I could no longer worry about the house being dusty, the laundry piling up, and the kids' next baseball practice. I now focused on me – in the short-term, on survival, in the longer-term, on living a long, healthy and fulfilling life! In the long run, life's everyday, mundane chores will not be a concern, so I set those aside. Other, generally more important concerns that may include family, career, economics, while more difficult, would also have to become secondary.

The moment I began to take an active stance toward my treatment and recovery was when I truly developed a strong sense of self-determination and control over my destiny. I focused every ounce of energy that I possessed into gathering information and learning in order to ensure I was making sound decisions. I bought books and literature, searched the internet, asked my physicians countless questions and constantly requested information of them (I'm certain I was driving them crazy!) I asked for charts, graphs, explanations, and recommendations. I insisted that my physicians make any medical jargon understandable to me. If I was to choose among various treatments, I would make certain that I knew exactly the potential demands (of me) and benefits of each, before moving forward. I needed to believe that the treatment would result in progress. I was an active participant in my treatment program. I felt in charge and still had much to do.

During my research I stumbled upon other potentially beneficial, albeit somewhat "different" forms of treatment. I found that I could integrate complementary modalities into my treatment plan and that each may play an important role in my long-term survival. I began to incorporate acupuncture, reflexology, colonics, proper nutrition, Eastern medicine, chiropractic care and therapeutic massage. These treatments helped to relieve the side effects of chemotherapy, strengthened my immune system, and perhaps most importantly, relieved stress. I firmly believe that the integration of these modalities with conventional medicine is essential for recovery, as they all contribute to strengthening body and mind alike. If it had not been for my active research, I would never have even considered any of these treatments. After doing so, I realized how important it can be to keep an open mind and consider all available options, when searching for the best cancer treatment plan. My personal, integrated treatment plan may not necessarily be what is best for everyone, but I believe that exploring all options is vitally important (and should be driven by that action-oriented attitude!) An open-minded approach can support the overall wellness of the mind, body, and spirit, which may materially improve the chances of recovery and long-term survival.

Positive thinking can help to achieve wellness, and an active approach to treatment which includes exhausting all options, can dramatically increase the chances of survival. Optimism and action go hand in hand in the battle against cancer. No matter how severe the diagnosis, I believe that recovery from cancer is a much stronger possibility if the patient marshals their inner power to think positively and to truly believe that everything they are doing in combination to "beat cancer" is working.

Cancer is not necessarily a death sentence. Whether cancer is discovered in its early stages, or has progressed to stage four, it is important to understand that the diagnosis is like being handed a road map of your future life — you need to study it and decide where and how you want to travel.

I have known and loved many strong individuals that sadly, have died from cancer. In contrast, there are also many cancer survivors — more and more each year. I am an ordinary person and I have survived the most terminal stage of breast cancer. The reality is that I am no more physically durable or strong-minded than any other person. I believe that we all possess the inner strength to fight cancer, and that God does not place challenges before us that He has not equipped us to handle. We all have the potential to harness that strength in order to face and overcome the obstacles that we encounter in our lives. If I can do it, I have faith that you can too!

Chapter 2

The Power of Early Diagnosis and Multiple Opinions

"Question the doctor – The lesson for a patient is to ask your doctor about treatment options, why they would or would not apply, and why a certain treatment is being recommended. Then, get another opinion from another type of doctor such as a radiologist or urologist who specializes…. and ask the same questions."

Hollister H. Hovey. "Too Quick To Cut."
The Wall Street Journal December 9, 2003

As mentioned in the previous chapter, a main component of an action-oriented attitude is an open mind that explores all options. Early detection and diagnosis and multiple opinions will direct and position you on a path of action.

This chapter will address a number of early warning signs that could help avoid cancer before it emerges or detect it in its earliest stages. Education can provide opportunities to recognize some early signs of cancer that could present as a painful lump in your breast, a chronic cough or a persistent watery eye. It could also possibly enable you to help another who is curious or worried about an irregularity or radical change in their health. Whether a friend, loved one, or acquaintance, you may be able to notice various indicators and advise on the importance of immediate examination by a physician. And, learning what the early signs are will help you better understand your own body's status.

Acquiring a second, and possibly third opinion, is often a key factor in surviving cancer. This chapter will explain the approach that I believe is the most productive based on my research and personal experience. It will address why multiple opinions are important and how to go about obtaining them.

Early Warning Signs and Detection. There are clinical procedures that can identify cancer: blood tests, mammograms, x-rays, physical examinations, biopsies, etc. Many of these methods will indicate whether or not cancer is a possibility. However, personal awareness of your body and its overall wellness and recognition of the signs it sends you, can be a powerful weapon in the battle against cancer. Understand that you are the most valuable asset to every endeavor in that battle. In my case, I was assured that there was no evidence of cancer in my body. However, not only did I have an egg-sized tumor in my breast, the cancer had spread throughout my lymphatic system and I had two tumors in my liver. If I had not persistently "listened" to what my body was "telling me" via the signs it was sending, then without a doubt, I would not be alive today.

Pay close attention to your body; it's constantly trying to make you aware of its status. The National Cancer Institute website lists a sampling of a wide variety of symptoms that cancer can cause:

- Thickening or lump in the breast or any other part of the body
- Obvious change in a wart or mole
- A sore that does not heal
- Nagging cough or hoarseness
- Changes in bowel or bladder habits
- Indigestion or difficulty swallowing
- Unexplained changes in weight
- Unusual bleeding or discharge

The site goes on to point out that when these symptoms occur, they are not always caused by cancer. They may also be signs of infections, benign tumors, or other problems. The point is, it is important not to ignore what your body is telling you and to see a doctor soon. One should not wait, as early cancer usually does not cause pain.

Diagnostic Methods and Potential Shortcomings. For the most part, conventional detection is effective but there are certain situations that have produced inaccurate results. Blood tests are one example. This form of detection is often successful but is not perfect. Blood tests are most beneficial in pinpointing the progression or regression of cancer, but have a tendency to distinguish material that is unrelated (to cancer) or caused by an entirely different illness.

This creates the possibility of a positive cancer diagnosis when it should have been negative. Conversely, there is also the danger of a negative diagnosis when in fact, cancer does exist. At the time of my diagnosis, my CA27.29 test fell within normal limits. This is a blood test that measures a substance that breast cancer cells secrete into the bloodstream. Some normal cells also make it, and some breast cancer cells do not secrete it at all. This was the case in my situation. Obviously, believing that you do not have cancer, when you actually do, can be fatal.

An incorrect diagnosis can also be made from mammograms. Typically, the breasts of women under age forty are denser than the breasts of older women. This makes it more difficult for mammograms to consistently detect cancer across women of all age groups. I discovered this the hard way. I wish I had known this when I had my first mammogram at age thirty-four. I believe this is one of the main reasons for my misdiagnosis. Fortunately, persistence led me to a more precise method of detection. I am thrilled that now pre-menopausal women have the option of digital mammography. It is helping identify tumors earlier.

Two years later, I received a proper diagnosis through biopsy. The **only sure way** to diagnose breast cancer is a biopsy. Other procedures simply hint at the possibility of cancer. In spite of this, a biopsy is not 100% accurate, even if it is the most effective diagnostic method. According to Colonel Craig Shriver, M.D., F.A.C.S., M.C., Director and Principal Investigator - Clinical Breast Care Project, Program Director and Chief - General Surgery Service of Walter Reed Army Medical Center, and Associate Professor of Surgery for the Uniformed Services University, "Eighty percent of all biopsies are negative, meaning they are benign or non-cancerous. If, in fact, a biopsy comes back positive, in my opinion, once diagnosed with breast cancer, even if non-invasive, the patient should obtain an opinion or evaluation at a comprehensive cancer center at that point. There are studies in medical literature supporting improved cancer survival outcomes, at certain "Centers of Excellence", especially for complex types of cancers or when multi-disciplinary treatment is given. These are very strictly defined organizations that are designated by the National Cancer Institute as having expertise in various types of cancers with regard to clinical and basic scientific research. This has been clearly shown for breast cancer, pancreatic cancer and rectal cancer."

Colonel Shriver also suggests one visit *www.oncolink.com*, as it is very user-friendly and under constant peer review. "It does not allow links or information that does not meet rigorous standards that most medical professionals desire. This site does the homework for the patients and should certainly be regarded as being the best information available."

Keep in mind that the diagnosis is only as good as the pathologist. Pathology is the medical specialty that reviews and studies biopsies to determine proper diagnosis. The pathologist's level of expertise is a key factor in the success of the procedure, so be certain to locate a Board-certified pathologist, specializing in oncology. The National Cancer Institute does rate and set strict criteria with regard to cancer centers and their "approved" physicians. According to Col. Shriver, the two best sources for obtaining this information are the National Cancer Institute website, *www.nationalcancerinstitute.com*, and also at the same site, one could research "SPORE" also known as "Specialized Program of Research Excellence" sites.

Multiple Opinions. The horrifying words "you have cancer" have a tendency to cause panic. These thoughts manifest in the hours and days following your diagnosis. Do not let them control your actions. You will need a clear head in order to obtain multiple opinions, and you should not attempt to do so in desperation or haste. A useful fact about cancer is that in most cases there is a sufficient amount of time to organize a qualified treatment team and an effective treatment program. The plan starts in your mind with "positive thinking" and execution of the plan begins with acquiring a second and possibly third medical opinion. A Wall Street Journal article by Hollister H. Hovey, dated December 9, 2003, states "More than 200,000 men will be diagnosed with prostate cancer in the U.S. this year, but despite a number of treatment options, many men will undergo a radical prostatectomy without considering other less invasive procedures that might be just as effective." One reason men diagnosed with prostate cancer obtain other opinions is that these patients are often referred to surgeons, whereas many newer treatments are performed by other physicians such as urologists, radiologists or oncologists who specialize in prostate malignancies. "Doctors have a great tendency toward *you've got cancer, take it out,*" says Peter Scardino, a surgeon and Chairman of the Department of Urology at New York's Memorial Sloan-Kettering Cancer Center.

I learned first-hand the importance of multiple opinions as I witnessed my brother Lance fight cancer. He was misdiagnosed for three years before he lost his battle to cancer at the young age of thirty-five. Lance was first diagnosed with a rare form of sarcoma. Chemotherapy was not effective for this type of cancer, so his physicians opted to surgically remove his tumors on four different occasions. Each time, the tumors returned. After a few years, a family friend (Thank you Cheryl!) suggested we consult with a team of physicians at M.D. Anderson Cancer Center in Houston, Texas. We had no knowledge of this facility, nor did we know what a comprehensive cancer center was. Within the first forty-eight hours there, we were told that Lance had a totally different kind of cancer — one that was generally very receptive to chemotherapy. Unfortunately, it was too late and my brother could not be saved.

While losing Lance was dreadfully hard to endure, it provided me with an experiential understanding that multiple pathology opinions are an absolute necessity. If not for Lance, I might have accepted my initial diagnosis and I would probably be gone now.

Obtaining multiple opinions is literally that important. While some may see this as directly questioning or challenging a physician's professional judgment, it is not — it is simply verifying the diagnosis and comparing more than one point of view. When it comes to life or death, forget about offending your physician. You need to find the best team of physicians to help you fight your cancer. That needs to become your new full-time job! You need to see one, two, even three physicians before you settle on a treatment plan. If two opinions match, you may have the facts you need to make a sound decision. If for any reason you don't feel 100% comfortable with what a physician is proposing, then obtain yet another opinion. It's your life.

Staging and Grading of Cancer. Staging or grading of cancer requires a series of examinations and testing which are conducted in order to learn the extent of the cancer. The same Wall Street Journal article quoted previously, also states, "Although the initial diagnosis of prostate cancer is generally correct, about 20% of the time mistakes are made in the staging and grading of the cancer, in a review of thousands of second opinions issued by researchers at John Hopkins School of Medicine in Baltimore." While the focus of this article is prostate cancer, it does underscore the importance of second opinions not only to determine the exact type of cancer, but also the extent of cancer in the body.

Staging of cancer is described by the NCI as "performing exams and tests to learn the extent of the cancer within the body, especially whether the disease has spread from the original site to other parts of the body. It is important to know the stage of the disease in order to plan the best treatment." For further information on staging and grading of cancer, visit the National Cancer Institute's website listed in the resource section of this book.

Choosing Your Physician(s). First, locate and consult a <u>board-certified</u> oncologist before undergoing any surgery. According to *HealthGrades.com*, "Board certified physicians have completed extensive training and testing, going above and beyond medical practice licensure. Each medical specialty has a national board responsible for setting standards that physicians must meet in order to be certified. Board certified physicians have completed several years of training beyond medical school, have practiced for a designated number of years in that specialty, and have passed examinations in their specialty area. Once certified, physicians must attend continuing medical education programs throughout their careers in order to remain certified. Some physicians have more than one board certification."

Dr. Shriver further clarifies: "Board-certification refers to a physician who has taken all the required training, and passed all of the rigorous requirements of the Hematology-Oncology Boards of the American Board of Medical Specialties (this applies only to Medical Oncologists in this regard). Surgical Oncologists should have completed training in a Society of Surgical Oncology-approved Fellowship Training Program, as there are no Boards available at this time for Surgical Oncologists."

Obviously, there is a significant difference between an oncologist and a general practitioner physician. An oncologist specializes in the treatment of cancer, and has received specialized, in-depth education and training, and therefore will have a greater understanding of what to expect from a given cancer diagnosis. A general practitioner is trained to treat a number of illnesses such as influenza, broken bones, sprains, separations, dislocations, fever, infection, etc. This type of practice requires a broad education of various types of illness and injury that is not typically concentrated in any one area such as cancer. You most certainly want a physician trained to recognize and treat your particular disease. Again, in my opinion, it is crucial that you meet with an oncologist prior to surgery.

Next, simply be aware that many physicians are connected to one another in a variety of ways. Subsequent opinions should not be impacted by a previous one. My research made it apparent that there is the possibility of a physician simply agreeing with a preceding opinion. I believe this is done to avoid conflict with another physician so as not to compromise their professional opinion. In order to prevent this from happening, you need to search for an oncologist who is not associated with the initial or former treating physician. It is likely easier to secure independent, unbiased opinions, if obtained at entirely different hospitals, even in different cities or states. If possible, try to avoid informing the oncologist of the original diagnosis or previous method of treatment until after their opinion has been provided. These steps will provide an unbiased point of view that can be more easily compared to other opinions.

While consulting a Board-certified oncologist helps to ensure your access to the high level of expertise you seek, it is also important for you to know the extent of his/her qualifications. Check their credentials. Ask what college and medical school they attended. Do they have knowledge of and access to clinical and experimental trials? Inquire about the extent of experience in the field of patient care in addition to that of their associates. When you choose an oncologist, they will be your partner throughout your cancer journey, so make certain you are confident in his/her abilities.

I obtained second and third opinions before making my final decision regarding which physicians to work with. I selected a multi-disciplinary team of physicians at M.D. Anderson Cancer Center in Houston, Texas. My oncologist, the pathologist, the team of surgeons (breast, liver and eye) and the radiologist all consulted with one another and with me, after reviewing all the tests and scans. This team of professionals informed and educated me about all of my options. As a team, they concluded that pre-operative chemotherapy offered me the greatest hope for survival. I felt comfortable with their level of combined expertise. The time and effort I expended searching for this team was well worth it.

Developing a Partnership With Your Physician. Your physician's communication skills can help you detect whether they will truly care and tend to your needs. The way they communicate with you and your family, can provide insight as to whether you are viewed as a patient or a project. You are entitled to a physician who attempts to build a relationship with you and considers your feelings and input important.

I recall a particular appointment in the very beginning of my journey when my husband and I went together to obtain another opinion. The physician explained to us that although he was sure it was nothing he would have to perform a biopsy to confirm that. It was encouraging that he was willing to take this precaution. However, when we asked if this procedure would leave a scar, he replied "yes" in a rude and demeaning tone of voice. We then asked if perhaps he could perform the procedure in such a way as to inflict a less noticeable scar, and he answered very rudely "NO!" We then felt silly for asking the questions. On the way home, my husband and I discussed the physician's attitude and decided that it would be best to seek yet another opinion from another physician before making our final decision. Bedside manner and how comfortable you feel during visits are very important when choosing your medical team.

Ensure the physician uses language that you and your family can understand. Do they make you aware of your options and take the time to help you understand them? Is your physician listening to your questions and willing to take the time to answer them? Do they ask you if what they've said is clear? Does your physician seem rushed and unfocused or attentive and caring? Are they making you aware of the fact that there are clinical trials underway for nearly all types of cancer? Take the time to consider all possible clinical trials that you may be eligible for.

Consider all treatment options offered to you. For instance, I was first told that traditional chemotherapy would most likely be of no benefit to me at my stage four diagnosis. It turned out that my lead oncologist at M.D. Anderson Cancer Center (and my MDACC team) highly recommended an experimental chemotherapy regimen – one which they felt offered hope. Had I opted for the traditional chemotherapy, it may have disqualified me from being accepted into the experimental protocol.

To this day, I feel blessed that I was able to participate in the Taxotere/Herceptin clinical trial in May of 2000. Nine years later, I continue to receive Herceptin infusions, a drug developed by a leading biotechnology research firm, Genentech, Inc., specifically for metastatic breast cancer in HER2 over-expressed tumors (for more information visit www.gene.com). It could be one of the reasons I am alive and well today!

Financial Considerations. Obtaining multiple opinions can be expensive. Insurance often does not cover all charges in this category. Do not allow financial considerations to hinder your chances of long-term survival. If money is a concern, seek a non-profit cancer foundation that can help guide you. The American Cancer Society has a great financial resource page. Check your local affiliate offices of national agencies. Your local agencies are typically a great help in finding resources available in your area. Do some research – be proactive. I found that it is possible to receive social security disability income if you have been diagnosed with (stage IV) cancer. The logic underlying provision of these benefits is that the Social Security Administration considers anyone diagnosed with life-threatening illnesses to be entitled to the funds they have paid in to the system over the years now, given the fact they may not live to retirement age. I urge you to research this possibility. It may prove to be of considerable financial assistance and help enable you to go wherever you need to in order to receive the best possible treatment.

Using what my family had learned throughout my brother's cancer journey, I chose to go to a Comprehensive Cancer Center. The best physicians are hired by facilities that have an outstanding reputation. Comprehensive Cancer Centers such as M.D. Anderson in Houston and DUKE in Raleigh-Durham only accept physicians with specialized expertise in the field of cancer. These physicians treat hundreds of cancer patients every month as opposed to every year.

Another important attribute of Comprehensive Cancer Centers was explained to me during my interview with my lead oncologist at M.D. Anderson. He said, "One of the advantages that we have here is our multi-disciplinary planning for new patients." He continued to explain, "Everybody puts their heads together and usually when you present a patient you can tell pretty well what the recommendations are going to be, but occasionally there are little wrinkles you don't think of and sometimes recognizing these wrinkles makes a big difference." He then gave an example of an event in which easily overlooked indicators or, "little wrinkles" were discovered. He explained, "A patient who we saw a few days ago had previously been treated for breast cancer and we had a very experienced breast surgeon who was able to explain why things went wrong (previously) based on his review of the scars from her previous breast surgery."

This particular example illustrates how multi-disciplinary planning for new patients serves to individualize each patient's treatment. The care given to the woman my oncologist referred to, was unique to her case. Her physicians at M.D. Anderson "put their heads together" in a successful effort to recognize and explain "little wrinkles" or indicators of faulty treatment she had received in the past so they could understand what was going wrong in the present and prevent further problems.

When I arrived at M.D. Anderson in April of 2000, my oncologist made me aware of certain treatment plans that probably would have been useless and possibly harmful. I had previously been told that surgery was required. If I had not sought multiple opinions, I would never have known that in my case, surgery would have been more harmful than beneficial, prior to my chemotherapy. Persistence saved me from making this huge mistake.

There were two reasons that I needed to be treated with chemotherapy before undergoing surgery. First, the tumor in my left breast had to be shrunk before it could be safely removed. Second, my preoperative chemotherapy was needed to kill a majority of cancer cells that existed throughout my lymphatic system and in my liver. The size of the lump in the breast can indicate the severity of breast cancer and sometimes help to "stage" the cancer. (My breast tumor was 7cm by 4cm, which is very large, and the extent of disease likely meant that my cancer had spread outside of its original location within my breast). Predominantly, surgery is performed to remove a portion of the body in which cancer originated. Cancer cells that may linger and move beyond their initial location, often "retaliate" by metastasizing more rapidly and occupying other vital organs in the body. My physicians at M.D. Anderson considered my oversized breast tumor as an indication that cancer cells had most likely spread outside of my breast. They administered preoperative chemotherapy in the hope of killing these straying cells. (Many tests were performed in advance and their suspicions were confirmed — as you might guess, the day I learned this was one of the worst days of my life.) My physicians gave many reasons for every action. More importantly, they personalized my individual treatment and for this, I will be forever grateful. I believe all cancer patients deserve highly individualized treatment as well. Settle for nothing less. Your expectations should be sky high when it is your life that it is in jeopardy!

In summary,

- Listen to your body and the signals it sends you.
- Obtain multiple opinions to ensure early and proper diagnosis.
- If possible, choose a hospital that specializes in your particular disease.
- Rely on your intuition and common sense.
- Be persistent and determined to find the best physician and a Comprehensive Cancer Center that best fits you and your current condition.
- Maintain your positive thinking throughout this venture, and
- Help as many people as you can along the way.

Believe. You will survive, you will prevail.

Chapter 3

The Power of Combining All Medicine

"I believe that the remedial options which exist outside of Western medical practice, should not be considered substitutes, but rather as complementary attributes of an integrated treatment program."

Throughout this book, I talk about certain forms of complementary medicine: acupuncture, reflexology, colonics, Eastern herbal medicine, proper nutrition, chiropractic care and therapeutic massage. These have been vital components of my treatment program and I personally, have never considered them to be "alternatives". The word "alternative" tends to imply that such remedies are located on the opposite end of the spectrum in comparison to conventional medicine. I believe that the remedial options which exist outside of Western medical practice, should not be considered substitutes, but rather as complementary attributes of an integrated treatment program.

The purpose of exhausting all treatment options is to seek all that is necessary to your survival, and potentially beneficial in relieving troublesome or painful side effects of certain types of treatment. Choose components which you and your physician believe will be the most effective, and combine them into a personalized treatment program. Then pursue each religiously, with an effort to recover and attain a state of wellness that demonstrates "no evidence of disease." Viewing Western and Eastern medicine in combination is an idea which I strongly urge you to consider.

If you have been diagnosed with cancer, Western medicine should be chosen first and foremost, before exploring complementary medicine. Keep in mind that like it or not, health care in the U.S. is big business. Most general physicians are well trained and truly want to do their best for their patients. However, in my experience, unless they are entirely convinced that they are unqualified to treat cancer patients, most doctors are unlikely to refer such patients to a comprehensive cancer center.

Once you have decided on a team that will administer your conventional treatment, you will have reached a point where you can extend your treatment program and supplement Western medicine by incorporating complementary modalities. If you can think of your total treatment plan as music, then complementary modalities are but a few strings that are played in order for the instrumental harmony of medicine to undulate closer toward perfection — they are neither inferior nor superior to Western medicine.

Complementary medicine does not deplore the deficiencies of conventional medicine; instead it intensifies the cause to find a cure and strengthens the effort to heal. In the same respect, my success thus far implies that Western medicine alone does not reign above all other medical practices. The fact that I combined other modalities with my conventional treatment and have survived the most advanced stage of cancer is what has fueled my belief that Western medicine can successfully incorporate complementary medicine in order to penetrate the glass ceiling of "terminal illness."

According to the mortality statistics relating to stage IV cancer, I was expected to live for eighteen months, beginning at the point of diagnosis; my chance of survival was three percent or less. Essentially what this means is that historically, Western medicinal practice and its demonstrated capabilities have not proven effective in curing such an advanced stage of illness. It has been nine years, I am still alive with no evidence of disease and my Western doctors cannot explain why, except for the occasional statement, "You have been very lucky."

It seems odd to me that a physician who specializes in the medical profession, an occupation that requires such precise science, would refer to a result as "luck." I am not aware of any "luck theory" that exists among scientific discovery or hypothesis. Science is a word that we use to label the pursuit of discovering the undiscovered, explaining the unexplained, and proving what has not yet been proven. In my opinion "luck" is a word that is used to label events and occurrences that science should be able to explain but unfortunately cannot. Conventional medicine remains an important and primary portion of my treatment yet the doctors who I chose to administer my treatment cannot clarify the reason I have been able to triumph over cancer. Obviously, within the realm of Western medicine and the scientific notions that apply, a certain amount of luck was involved in my survival which basically equates to the uncertainty of why I am still alive and in what currently appears to be a disease-free state.

This confusion among my doctors is not a result of incompetence or inexperience. On the contrary, I believe that the doctors I chose were extraordinarily qualified and through my survival, their expertise undoubtedly precedes them. They have mastered the art of Western medicine. However, it is my belief that the abundant education that they acquired within this practice has ironically, reduced their ability to understand and explain my recovery. In order to specialize in the field of cancer all of their focus had to be directed upon the teachings of Western medicine. They were not required to educate themselves about the benefits of complementary modalities. Their understanding is limited in regard to the treatment I pursued outside of the conventional boundaries in which they practice. When they ponder the reason for my survival they only think in terms of what they know and have studied and do not consider factors (such as complementary medicine) of which their knowledge is impartial. Therefore, when I hear the word "luck" spoken by my doctors, in my mind it translates as a lack of understanding the potential benefits of integrating complementary medicine in order to strengthen or broaden the reach of Western medicine.

There are three main procedures that are used in Western medicine to combat cancer: surgery, radiation and chemotherapy. In a surgical operation, a tumor or section of the body where tumors are located is removed. Radiation therapy is the use of ionizing radiation to shrink tumors or kill cancer cells. Chemotherapy is the use of cytotoxic chemicals meant to kill cancer cells. Biological therapies are showing more promise as a fourth procedure. (See Chapter 10) Hormone therapy and stem cell transplantation are therapies also used in treating some types of cancer. The National Cancer Institute web site has comprehensive information on all of these procedures.

Surgery. Surgery is considered a local therapy designed to remove the tumors and surrounding tissues. Again, I emphasize the importance of asking questions and obtaining multiple opinions **before having surgery**. Fear sometimes drives the decision to just cut "it" out…meaning "get the cancer out of my body!" Consider all of your treatment options prior to having any procedure. Surgery is invasive and recovery time is unique to the procedure and the individual. The body heals best in a relaxed state, so remember to give yourself the quiet time you need to heal fully.

Radiation. I have not received radiation as part of my cancer journey. I mention it because it is one of Western medicine's three most common treatments for cancer. Radiation can be used alone to treat cancer or used in conjunction with other therapies. The most commonly used radiation therapy is external and is usually an outpatient procedure. Internal radiation can require a hospital stay. There are different types of radiation for different cancers. A highly skilled team creates the radiation treatment plan for each patient. One of the most important steps in the design of an individual's treatment plan is the simulation. This helps the team deliver the most precise, efficient treatment while protecting healthy tissues as much as possible. Skin care is important for the radiation "field." Basically your skin appears to be getting sunburned. I have referred emu oil to many of my friends who have received radiation and I was told it helped immensely! Ask your doctor for suggestions about what to do to keep your skin healthy.

Chemotherapy. According to Col. Shriver, "In some patients it would appear that chemotherapy kills, if not all breast cancer cells that are out there somewhere waiting to continue to grow in the future, it kills enough of them so that the body's immune system can take over and kill the rest of the cells." You benefit from chemotherapy's ability to destroy cancer cells, but it may not kill all cancer cells present and in its attempt to do so it will also kill your good white blood cells or T-cells. White blood cells are your body's natural defense against disease. Therefore, chemo drastically decreases the effectiveness of your immune system. On this topic Col. Shriver states, "We definitely know that the immune system plays a role in keeping cancers in check or preventing them from spreading… it's a very complex interplay between the cancer, the body's immune system, the person, the genetics, the environment, the diet."

Having a strong immune system is important and complementary modalities place significant emphasis on strengthening the immune system. While chemo kills the cancer cells, complementary modalities can be employed to reinforce the body's natural immunity, providing the body the ability to attack disease (thereby complementing chemo's ability to kill cancer cells). We will discuss ways I have changed my diet in order to improve the quality of my immune system later in the book.

Col. Shriver openly expresses the great importance of the body's immune system in the survival of cancer: "…the truth of the matter is, we don't know in an individual patient whether it is going to work — to kill all or enough of the cancer cells, so that the immune system can take over and do the rest of the job and prevent cancer from coming back in the future." I interpret his statement to mean that the immune system needs to be strong if you are going to survive. Complementary medicine can be incorporated into your overall treatment specifically for this purpose.

Proper nutrition in conjunction with IsAgenix cellular cleansing, acupuncture, chiropractic care, therapeutic massage, reflexology, and colonics, are all complementary modalities which I believe have dramatically strengthened my immune system. I know that these therapies, combined with my conventional treatment have worked hand in hand, to contribute to my survival. I feel that if you believe and are committed to your treatment plan and your overall journey back to optimal health and wellness, you too, can achieve the same result.

Chapter 4

The Power of Acupuncture

"It is time to ambush and surround your illness by employing every possible modality that can potentially attack cancer cells."

Acupuncture is a word that many people recognize but are often uncertain as to what it really is. This form of therapy is growing rapidly in popularity in the United States. However, it has not been a commonly accepted form of treatment in our cultural history. The majority of our country's medical practices consist of Western medicine, although the benefits of complementary Eastern remedies are becoming more widely understood, bolstered by the testimony of those who have experienced their healing power.

Every year there is more empirical evidence to support the effectiveness of acupuncture. Recently a study was released by the Henry Ford Hospital Radiation Oncology Department showing that acupuncture can help relieve hot flashes in breast cancer patients. I believe it successfully supplemented my conventional treatment in such a way that leads me to stress the importance of its consideration and possible trial.

As discussed in the prior chapter, treatment is often more successful when highly individualized, and it is possible that acupuncture may not be the best option for you. That being said, I ask you to keep an open mind, realize that you could possibly benefit from acupuncture, and avoid the tendency to rely solely upon a Western treatment regimen. It is time to ambush and surround your illness by employing every possible modality that can potentially attack cancer cells. There is no doubt that our culture has made fantastic strides in health care in general, and much has been learned about cancer and how to combat it in the past fifty years. However, I believe that to view our Western treatments as superior, or as your only option, is off base. As you know, there is a vast world that exists beyond the United States, and there are various treatments that have existed in some cases, for thousands of years, in cultures that extend far beyond our own country's borders. Please do not dismiss these treatments simply because they seem strange or unfamiliar. Acupuncture could indeed prove to be a valuable ally in your fight against cancer.

In reality, many forms of conventional treatment rely on concepts that are similar to the ideology that acupuncture is based upon. Some of the most technological and scientific Western modalities are administered according to and based on the flow of energy that exists in our bodies. Acupuncture seeks to manipulate these currents of energy so as to relieve pain, stress, inflammation, nausea, fatigue, etc. The usefulness of acupuncture as it relates to cancer is that among other benefits, it can greatly reduce the side effects of chemotherapy. The very ailments that acupuncture can alleviate are coincidentally, some of the drawbacks of conventional treatment.

I promote the complementary use of acupuncture because it has proven to be beneficial throughout the duration of my cancer journey. However, I will not go as far as to say that acupuncture be seriously considered by every cancer patient, as it simply may not fit everyone's personality and/or beliefs. I have written this book with the intention of helping anyone with cancer and so, if acupuncture assists only one reader, then I will have achieved my goal. You may be that person. I challenge you to consider this option. There is of course, no guarantee that acupuncture will work for you and meet your approval. I only know that it is worthy of my praise, and that many others have experienced its effectiveness. It merits consideration and experimentation since it offers possible relief of painful and troublesome side effects. A dear friend of mine incorporated acupuncture as part of her treatment plan. She was able to play tennis up until one month prior to her death. I believe that acupuncture can help improve the quality of life for some cancer patients, and that, to me, is invaluable.

What is Acupuncture? Yes, acupuncture involves the insertion of needles into the skin. However, if one can look beyond that physical act, one will see that acupuncture is far more. Acupuncture has often been misunderstood. It is a medical practice that has been studied for centuries and mastered by Chinese and Japanese medicine men and women known as Shamans. The treatment can be traced back to ancient China, with the first records implying its use, being dated to 1600 B.C. It has survived the centuries and continually progressed to its current 21st century form. There is a reason that it has been around for so long and continues to be used. Through the ages, acupuncture has been proven to be an effective and therefore, valued form of healing.

While acupuncture is not necessarily included in the protocol of Western medicine, its use was approved by the Federal Drug Administration (FDA) in the early 1990s. The FDA recognized it to be beneficial in relieving pain and nausea especially among cancer patients receiving chemotherapy. This alone demonstrates that Western medicine practitioners in the United States are becoming increasingly aware of and comfortable with what acupuncture has to offer.

Understanding how and why acupuncture works will allow you to make a sound decision as to whether or not it may be of value as part of your total treatment plan. While I am not a qualified professional in the practice of acupuncture, I have researched its basic concepts and directly experienced its power. I found that besides strengthening my immune system to help combat cancer cells, it also greatly reduced the side effects of my chemotherapy.

You don't have to be an expert to understand the basic concepts of acupuncture. The main concept of acupuncture involves the manipulation of energy, that is, the flow of energy that is constantly pulsing throughout our bodies. These currents flow up and down pathways that are known as meridians, which are located on each side of the body and extend vertically from head to toe, and limb to limb. There are a total of twenty meridians, twelve being principal and eight that are secondary. Each meridian is unique and is associated with a certain organ such as the liver, heart, lung, intestine, or with an organ system such as the nervous, respiratory, digestive, or excretory system, etc. Meridians are the channels that carry our inner life force.

This notion of a "map" of meridians is quite possibly a new concept to you. If you are doubtful or disbelieving, then consider the basics of science and biology. We are well aware that everything tangible on this earth contains energy. Whether it is a human being or a pencil you write with, all matter contains a certain degree of energy. The human body binds an enormous energy flow. Consider this: by splitting a simple atom, Einstein was able to create an overload of energy powerful enough to destroy a large geographic area. Every cell in our bodies contains atoms which are composed of protons, neutrons, and electrons. This is energy in its smallest form. The main component of what can be the most powerful manifestation of energy can be found in your body, in each and every one of your cells.

Our main source of energy exists in our brain and nervous system. The brain encodes and decodes messages that are transported by our neuron cells to the part of the body that will carry out the particular function that each message transmits. Our neuron cells extend throughout our entire body and the impulses that they carry are electronic, which produces the constant flow of energy that travels through our body. Acupuncture uses this energy to heal and strengthen.

Consider this: a person is not entirely dead if his/her heart stops beating. Death is clinically pronounced when brain activity ceases — when the source of the energy flow is no longer functioning or producing energy. Your heart beat can be revived, although this is often accomplished by administering an electrical shock that basically jumpstarts your heart and does so through the use of energy.

The nutrients in the food we consume are used for energy to power the body. Again, we'll discuss more about how I continue to fuel my body later in the book. Our brain and nervous system uses this energy to transmit the involuntary and voluntary functions of the rest of the body. Involuntary refers to the functions of your organ systems and voluntary functions generally consist of the movements and actions that you make of which you are immediately aware. These functions result in the depletion of energy which leads to the need for replenishment. The overall result is that our bodies feed off energy, produce more energy, and release energy in a repetitive and continual process in order to survive. Anything that facilitates or strengthens this process, greatly contributes to one's overall wellness.

Acupuncture strives to increase as well as suppress, or sedate energy, in order to create a balance in its flow. Certain currents of energy in the human body will go "haywire" or be weakened, usually as a result of external factors such as stress. Acupuncture is a process that either tranquilizes energy that is out of control, or stimulates the flow of energy that has become exhausted. This is done by the insertion of thin needles into acupoints located along the meridians described earlier. There are over a thousand acupoints corresponding to the energy body. Each point exists as either a strengthening or sedating point. The needles are inserted millimeters beneath the skin and serve to either interfere with the flow of energy in order to slow its overflow, or stimulate the current of energy to increase its volume. Once again, meridians are the paths of energy that relate to various parts of the body that energy is flowing to, and acupoints indicate where each needle should be placed in accordance with each meridian.

An excess of energy or lack thereof can dramatically increase stress, both mentally and physically. Stress is a factor that can have a very significant and negative impact on one's mental attitude, immune system, and overall wellness. It has been proven that stress is a main cause of illness and I believe that it had a direct effect on the origins of my cancer. Stress seems to feed upon the imbalance it causes in the body and becomes stronger, more intense and increasingly difficult to bear.

Chemotherapy produces side effects that typically increase stress. Fatigue, nausea, and pain are dangerous stressors that decrease one's overall wellness. Acupuncture can relieve these ailments and in doing so, it will reduce stress which in turn, strengthens your immune system and empowers it to better fight cancer cells. While chemotherapy may kill cancer cells, at the same time it is poisoning your body and depleting its natural capabilities to combat cancer. Wellness equates with immunity. Therefore, if acupuncture can strengthen the immune system, it can serve as a beneficial complement to conventional medicine. I encourage you to research and experiment with acupuncture so that you can make an informed decision as to whether it is an appropriate complementary treatment for you.

Should you choose to try acupuncture, approach it in a manner similar to that described in the earlier chapter about seeking multiple opinions. Consider the following:

- Investigate the credentials of the acupuncturist. Ensure that they are qualified to administer the treatment. If not, then move on to another practitioner or ask a member of your treatment team for a recommendation. I found a qualified individual through a referral from my nutritionist. And of course, bedside manner is very important. Be certain you trust and feel comfortable with every member of your "wellness team".

- Discuss the manner in which treatment is administered. Chances are this is a new procedure for you. You will want your practitioner to be forthcoming with a description of the process so you will know exactly what to expect. As with any clinical procedure, sterility is of the utmost importance. All of the needles should be sterile and disposable. When you receive a vaccination, the area to be injected is sterilized (usually with alcohol); your acupuncturist should do the same.

- Inquire as to the short and long-term cost. Usually the cost will depend on the frequency and duration of the treatments. Prior to agreeing to treatment, consult your insurance company in order to learn the extent of coverage they will provide for you, if any.

Do not be afraid of offending the practitioner by asking these questions. This form of treatment is highly personalized and focused on the comfort of the patient. Your inquiries will most likely be well accepted. You in turn, will be asked numerous questions on your first appointment, in an effort to gather medical information about you as an individual and as a patient, so that the treatment can be conducted most effectively. The flow of energy is affected by wellness, lifestyle, and behavioral patterns and these are naturally different for each person. Therefore, each patient's acupuncture treatment varies according to their unique condition or state of wellness.

My own instincts compelled me to research other modalities in order to achieve overall success in my fight against cancer. If I had not incorporated complements such as acupuncture, I do not believe I would be alive and in good health today. While conventional treatment contributed a great deal to my recovery, it was interesting to witness my physicians' astonishment, confusion, and inability to understand or explain how I was improving so rapidly. My conventional physicians (i.e., practicing Western medicine) eventually realized how beneficial it was for me to integrate other forms of medicine into my wellness program.

In my opinion, complementary medicine is essential to your treatment. It provides integration and balance that can assist in fighting cancer. An integrated approach can bring you closer to perfection in terms of your treatment, and acupuncture can be a valuable part of your overall plan. Use this treatment time to incorporate visualization into your wellness program — picture yourself whole and well, progressing along the triumphant path of your cancer journey. Imagine that the acupuncture needles are arrows penetrating cancer cells in your body, and visualize those evil cells being destroyed! Strive to strengthen your immune system and achieve overall wellness. If acupuncture proves to be beneficial to you and if you believe in its effectiveness, then you will be one step closer to your long-term, disease-free survival.

Chapter 5

*The Power of Proper Nutrition
And IsAgenix*

*"Why do Western women have more breast cancer than
Eastern/Asian women? The answer seems to be in the diet.
That is a choice... processed foods, foods that are high in things
that lead to increased estrogen levels in women, increased
obesity which also increases the risk of breast cancer because
it increases circulating estrogen levels... these are lifestyle
choices."*

Col. Craig Shriver, M.D., F.A.C.S., M.C.

"You are what you eat..." I'm sure you've heard this phrase once
if not a thousand times, along with other sayings such as, "eat to
live, don't live to eat" or "your body is a temple." For some, especially
those who are healthy, or think they are healthy, these phrases may
seem trite, but they hold significant meaning: what we put into our
bodies has a direct effect on how much energy we can produce.

Proper nutrition and supplementation is vital to your health.
When you are fighting cancer, your survival depends upon your
overall wellness, which in turn is driven in large part by nutrition.
Question your physician if they tell you, "Go ahead and eat what

you want, enjoy your life while you still can." At the time I was diagnosed with stage IV cancer, several of my many physicians said this to me. I am very grateful that I chose not to take this advice. I wasn't about to bow down to cancer by thinking, "I am going to enjoy my life until my illness takes it from me." Instead, I planned to defeat cancer by empowering my mind and body to fight it. Simple common sense and logic helped me to realize that an enormous component of "living well" is "eating well."

When you are diagnosed with cancer, it's so easy to "comfort" yourself with foods that seem to "feed" emotional needs. For example, we're all familiar with how some people develop cravings for chocolate, something akin to an emotional attachment. Chocolate is even thought of as an "aphrodisiac." I'm sure you have heard someone say, "I have a bit of a sweet tooth." A person may be a chocolate lover or enjoy dessert after each meal, but this is not due to heredity or genetics. A "sweet tooth" is nothing more than an attachment to sweet foods that develops as a result of consistently eating dessert foods that are high in unnatural sugar. But cancer patients beware — cancer is fueled by eating sugar and foods that turn to sugar when consumed – NO MORE SUGAR.

Upon gaining extra weight, many people go on fad diets, or even fast. In many cases, people have success with these methods and drop the excess weight. Unfortunately, the majority eventually gain back the pounds. If you are among this group, and you plot the fluctuation of your weight on a timeline, you may find that your body weight has been rising and falling sporadically. This inconsistency will not help you to achieve the balance and tranquility needed for optimal wellness. Cancer causes disorder and chaos within your body. In order to survive, you must restore your body's equilibrium.

A large portion of balancing nutrition lies in maintaining a healthy, natural body weight. Obviously, some people naturally have a larger percentage of body fat than others. If you believe you are overweight, don't focus on shedding pounds. If you see yourself as overly thin, don't concentrate on gaining weight. Instead, if you direct your effort solely at proper nutrition, your body weight will gradually approach a natural, healthy level for you. In practicing proper nutrition, you are not dieting, you are not fasting, and you are not overeating; rather, you are simply consuming and absorbing the appropriate vitamins, minerals and nutrients your body needs in order to function at its peak.

My cancer diagnosis forced me to change my lifestyle. Eating well is a matter of knowing exactly what it is you are consuming and how it affects your bodily functions and overall health. Properly fueling your body requires knowing how and when you should eat certain foods and drink certain liquids.

It may be helpful to consult with a holistic nutritionist who can help you design a personalized nutrition plan to help support your body's immune functions and other natural rhythms. My nutritionist's guidance was invaluable in that it provided me with recommendations for healthful food choices, an all-natural vitamin and mineral supplementation program, and education on the elimination of toxins in my life that could tax and overburden my immune system.

The human body's immune system is an intricate network of specialized tissues, organs, cells and chemicals. The lymph nodes, spleen, bone marrow, thymus gland, and tonsils all play a role in fighting off germs and illnesses. When the immune system is functioning well, it is able to neutralize potentially infectious organisms before an infection can develop. The immune system also looks for cells in the body that could "morph" into cancerous cells and attempts to eradicate them.

Although diet and lifestyle both play a crucial role in maintaining a healthy immune system, equally important are immune-regulating herbs and supplements. Of course, many people can benefit from immune-balancing herbs and supplements, but those with cancer or other illnesses or allergies, are likely to benefit most.

I talked with cancer survivors and took my nutritionist's advice. Together, we developed a nutritional plan designed to help me combat cancer. Before my diagnosis, I made an effort to stay healthy by attempting to include the five food groups in each meal. As a cancer patient, I now realize that generally, much of what we've been taught about nutrition is not entirely accurate.

The body absorbs the vitamins, minerals and nutrients that it needs and passes on whatever is left as waste. This complex process requires energy. Different foods require the digestive system to use diverse amounts of energy. Protein, for example, takes more time and energy to digest than carbohydrates, while fruits take the least amount of time and energy. Your body can digest and put to use only two types of food at one time. You can benefit from a protein and a starch, but if you add a vegetable then one of the food groups will go to waste. In other words, the advantage of combining all five food groups at one meal is a myth. By eating five food groups in one sitting, basically, you are consuming more food than the body can handle. Only a portion of that food is actually used beneficially, the rest is stored as fat, passed through as waste, or collected as putrefaction along the walls of the colon. Instead of attempting to fit all five food groups into three full meals a day, focus on eating two food groups within five balanced, smaller meals, at least two hours apart, each day.

In the mornings I focus solely on eating foods that will alkalinize my body. Alkalinity is measured on the pH scale. The pH scale goes from 0 to 14 with 7 being neutral. Below 7 is acidic and above 7 is alkaline. Basically, alkalinizing provides an oxygen rich environment in my body to promote optimal healing. According to my nutritionist, an "alkaline body" is one nurtured with fresh fruits and vegetables - eaten raw, steamed or juiced - and purified water filtered by reverse-osmosis if possible. For a handy food alkalinity chart compiled by Dr. Russell Jaffee follow this link to the downloadable chart: *http://www.perque.com/who-we-are.asp.*

While drinking water should be continual throughout each day, fruit is most beneficial when consumed before noon. Fruit is digested faster than carbohydrates or proteins and should not be combined with any other food group. I would not recommend that fruit be mixed with any substance other than water. If the body is digesting a protein and fruit is consumed, the fruit will be passed quickly with little benefit. The protein is fully absorbed but the fruit goes to waste.

Combine portions of fruit with a few glasses of purified water. Do not drink tap water. If you do not have a water purifier then if possible, have one installed. Another option would be bottled water but you must be careful which brand you choose to purchase. My nutritionist recommended that I drink what she described as reverse osmosis water or distilled water. Whether you choose to install a purifier or purchase bottled water, make certain that you are consuming water that is as untainted and as decontaminated as possible.

It is recommended that a person drink at least eight glasses of water a day. At the height of my chemo treatments I was trying to drink twenty glasses of water over the course of a day. What's important is that you make a conscious effort to evenly hydrate your body each day.

Water should be your number one source of liquid, the second being green, red or white tea. If you drink any fruit juice, I recommend that it be freshly squeezed or juiced. At the grocery store, the foods and liquids sold in cans, jugs, bottles etc. are generally processed and filled with unnatural preservatives. Besides, when is the last time you treated yourself to freshly squeezed orange juice?

In the afternoon and evening you can focus on consuming proteins, vegetables and carbohydrates. Some good sources for protein would be: beans, seeds and raw, unsalted nuts. Try to avoid grilled meat cooked by gas or charcoal that can contain carcinogens. Eating raw or lightly steamed vegetables provides your body with an abundance of nutrients. Raw or steamed broccoli, carrots, brussel sprouts, asparagus, peas, would be great choices for afternoon or evening meals. Eat a steamed vegetable along with a protein and you have yourself a perfectly healthy and "properly combined" meal. Remember, your body processes foods like white bread, white pasta, and white rice more quickly into sugar (which fuels cancer).

Following the recommendations of my nutritionist and being pro-active in my own research has helped me keep my body healthy and my mind focused on wellness. My wellness plan evolves as my body's needs change. The key is having a plan that reduces stress about proper nutrition and that supports your body in its fight against cancer!

Note: I personally have found taking Noxylane, or AHCC (Alpha Hexose Correlated Compound), high-powered mushroom supplements, to be very beneficial. I have now been taking them for over eight years and in spite of all the chemo I have endured, I feel these have helped keep my immune system strong. By encouraging the development of large numbers of highly active granules within the NK (natural killer) cells, mushroom compounds work to "tune up" the immune system while optimizing T, B, and NK cell function. Published studies have shown mushrooms to increase NK cell activity by more than 300%, B cell activity by 250% or greater, and T cell activity by 200% better than other vitamin, herbal or medicinal mushroom therapies. For more information regarding these supplements, log onto *www.lanelabs.com.*

The Power of Cellular Cleansing with ISAGENIX. Since being diagnosed with a terminal illness at the age of 36, I am proud to say that I am here today, in a body that is whole and well! I have officially been diagnosed as "no evidence of disease" for the last seven years! Others who are newly diagnosed want to know what I do to maintain my state of health and wellness.

At the time of my diagnosis, in spite of a dire prognosis I embraced the best of all worlds; clinical trials and the best Western and Eastern modalities had to offer including acupuncture, therapeutic massage, chiropractic care, reflexology and colonics. My holistic nutritionist suggested I take a variety of herbs and supplements. Those added to the Chinese and Tibetan herbs I was taking meant swallowing 120 + pills or capsules a day. In my opinion, everything was working in harmony and my body was striving to once again reach a high level of wellness where illness could not exist.

My journey has not been a cake-walk and it is still not over. I have dedicated the last nine years to obtaining optimal health and wellness. Over the last year or so my original routine of supplementation started to feel burdensome to my body and immune system. Unfortunately, my body, after about eight years could not continue to swallow and process this huge number of supplements and vitamins. I knew I had to continue taking care of myself, but I desperately needed a change.

I had made a promise at the lowest point in my cancer journey to help others who are newly diagnosed – I believe the many twists and turns in my path over the course of the last nine years has helped me do this. My journey to wellness is ever evolving and with each turn I evaluate what is working, what feels right and if I need to make a change. While the nutritional and supplementation program outlined in the beginning of this chapter has served me well, change was needed.

Cellular Nourishment and Cleansing. At about this time, in February, 2008 a fellow survivor, Sara Bruckshaw, told me about a scientifically - based cellular nourishing and cleansing system. Once again, something was brought to me at the time in my cancer journey when it was truly needed! After Sara told me about these masterfully crafted products that work in harmony throughout our entire body, I couldn't wait to try IsAgenix. I cannot help but wonder how much simpler my journey back to optimal health and wellness may have been had this regimen existed when I was diagnosed in the year 2000. Hindsight is always better and my journey has been just as it was supposed to be. And, I am thrilled we have it now! I truly believe our bodies are the miracle – IsAgenix may just help guide our body in the right direction!

Although we cannot control the air we breathe, or the many pesticides and hormones we eat, we can choose what we nourish our bodies with. We can choose what we eat and drink. Even being diagnosed as terminal I am not 100% perfect all the time, after all, we are only human. What I can do is alkaline my cells, so illness cannot thrive in my body. That is my realistic goal.

For me, Western medical treatment and my triple doses of Herceptin every 21 days continue and probably will for the rest of my life. (Thanks again Genentech!) I am thrilled I am able to stay connected with survivors regularly via the Touched By Cancer

Foundation. But, for many who "finish" treatment I can see the fear in their eyes and feel the terror in their voice, *"What do I do now?"* is always the big question. Now, as I have stated throughout this entire book, I am not a doctor, I am only a patient that has lived, breathed, and survived a terminal cancer diagnosis. But in my opinion if we feed and nourish our bodies and cleanse every one of our 70 trillion cells on a regular basis, as living, breathing humans, I believe IsAgenix to be the best system available internationally. With people like Jack Canfield (**Chicken Soup for the Healthy Soul**) and Dr. John Gray (the **Mars/Venus** author) giving this nutritional and cellular cleansing system their "seal of approval" I feel honored to join them along with many others and refer it to everyone I meet who is striving and frantically searching for optimal health and wellness.

So, when is the right time to begin a nutritional cleansing program? Only you can decide. I reviewed my nutritional plan and have tweaked it to include the IsAgenix products. For instance, I have an IsaLean shake in the morning along with a vitamin and mineral loaded shot of Ionix Supreme. This line of products fulfills my supplemental requirements while drastically reducing the number of pills I take each day. Starting my day with a balanced combination of protein, carbohydrates, and healthy fats shifts part of the nutrition plan I began my journey with but I still felt change was needed. It did not take long for my body to respond to the new regimen of super-foods I was introducing. My body tells me by 10 AM or so if I am off schedule!

The IsAgenix shakes are amazing. I love this stuff! Even just after a week my body began craving them! I blend mine in the Isa Blender along with ice, water, IsaFruit and fresh fruit. I can truly feel it nourishing my body with the active enzymes. I have also just recently discovered Dr. John Gray's Mars/Venus shake for women and do not believe it could ever taste any better! Full of vitamins, minerals and nutrients, I rarely miss a day of having one or two shakes. IsAgenix provides me with a system that nourishes as well as cleanses my system on a cellular level. The cleansing protocol is not recommended for anyone who is pregnant, on active chemo or radiation or on blood thinners or anti-seizure medications. Full details on cleansing and the benefits of the entire IsAgenix product line are provided when starting the program.

My family and my friends are amazed at the transformation my body has taken since incorporating IsAgenix into my health and wellness plan. I am at my weight from high school, over 25 years ago and can honestly say I have never felt better. The main message I am trying to convey is to go with the flow, when your daily "regimen" starts feeling hard to do or out of balance, consider new ways to nourish your body. For me the answer is IsAgenix. I recommend you give it a try!

For complete information on the IsAgenix nutritional cleansing program visit: www.johnlober.isagenix.com. If you are interested feel free to e-mail me at LoriLober@aol.com or phone me at 816-589-2333.

Other resources for nutritional information that I have found helpful:

Dr. Tony O'Donnell CNC www.radiantgreens.com
and www.foodmatters.tv

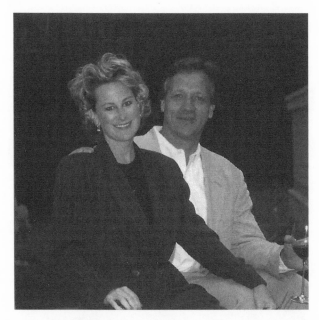

Summer 1995. My husband John and me. Our first summer together! One of my favorite photos "pre-cancer." Life was great!

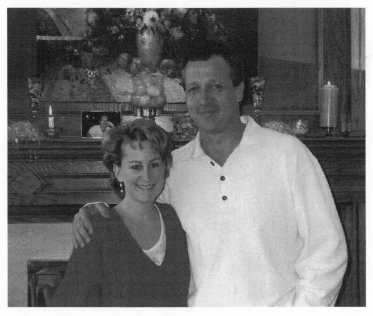

Easter 1996. John is my Prince Charming and the love of my life!

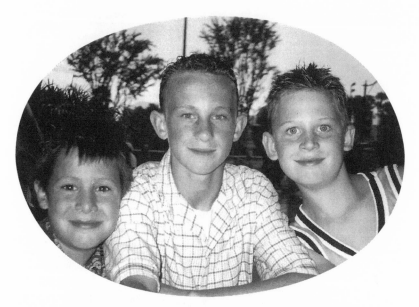

Summer 2000. John's sons, Danny and Anthony with Colby (in the center). So much to live for!

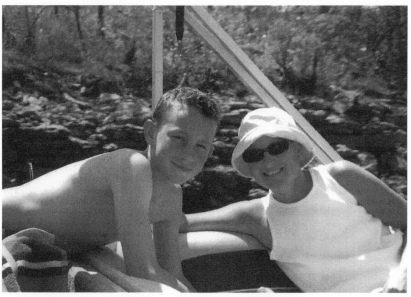

Labor Day Weekend 2000. With Colby; three weeks prior to the experimental radio-frequency ablation on my liver tumors at M. D. Anderson Cancer Center. How can this be happening to us?

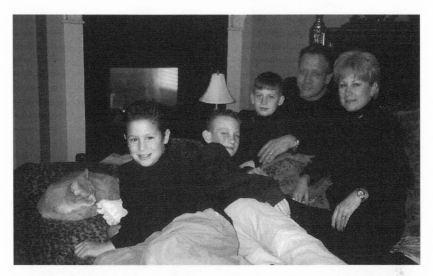

Christmas 2000. Smiles that Christmas were few and far between. We still did not know what to expect.

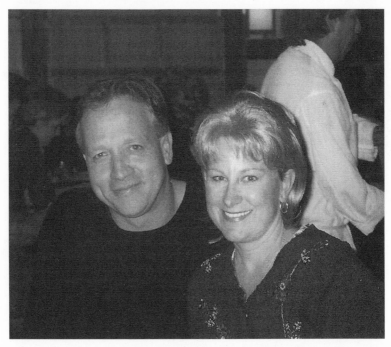

New Year's 2001. At The Hibachi on The Country Club Plaza in Kansas City, Missouri. My favorite place to eat! We always seem to meet our friends there! (Boy, was that wig bad!)

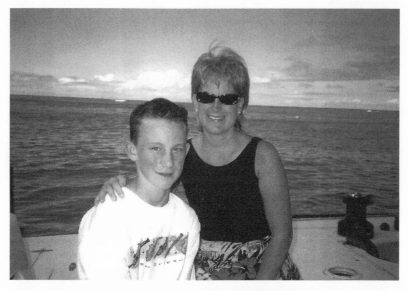

2001. In Oahu with Colby and another bad wig.

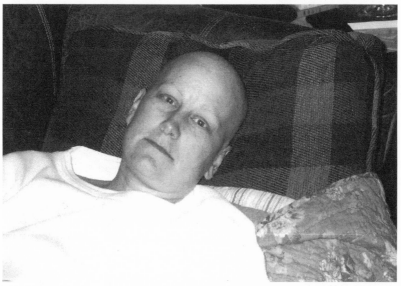

*Spring 2001. At times I just had to sleep. I couldn't eat, I couldn't talk, the
mouth sores were just too painful.*

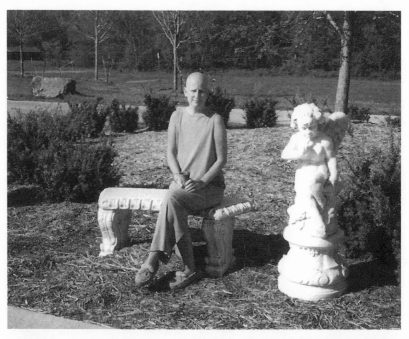

I prayed to my angels every day many, many times. "Was I going to live?"

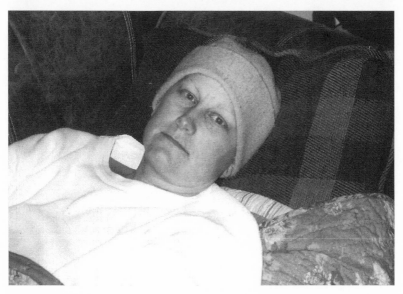

I still can't believe this is going on -- this was not part of any fairytale I had ever read.

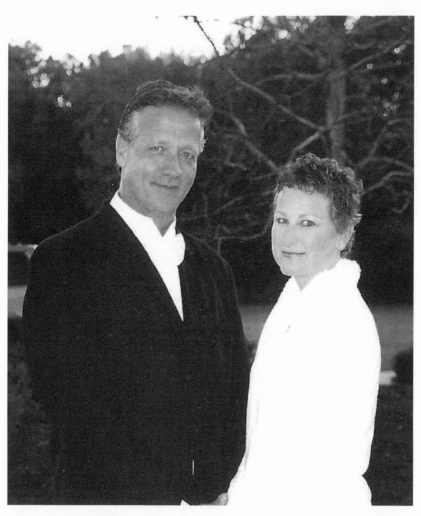

September 2001. Renewing our wedding vows. My hair was starting to grow back! The Shou Wu Wan was really working! We shared the special day with our closest friends! I was beginning to feel more optimistic about my journey.

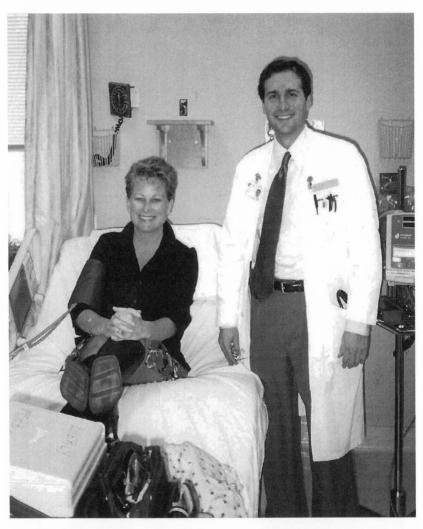

Spring 2002. With Dr. Michael Morse. I participated in an Immunization study at Duke in Durham, North Carolina. What a gift to be part of that trial! DUKE will forever be a beautiful part of my cancer journey!

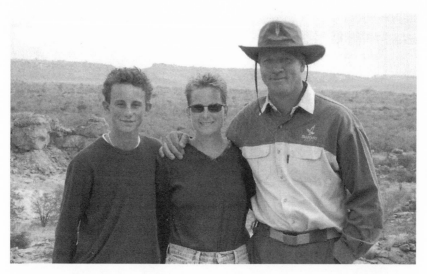

Summer 2002. John's dream trip of a lifetime to Zimbabwe to celebrate his 45th birthday! I was feeling better for the first time since April, 2000. I began "Bigger Than Pink" while he and Colby hunted the Plains game!

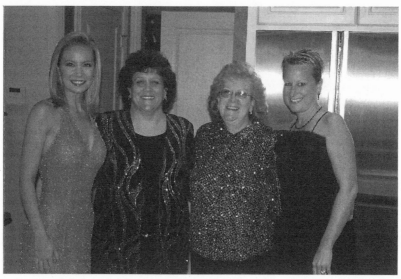

October 2002. First Show Home. Katie Harman, Miss America 2002, her mother, Darla Harman, my mom, Linda Wittmeyer and me! Having Katie to convey our foundation's message of hope and awareness across the nation has been one of my dreams come true! Thank you Katie!

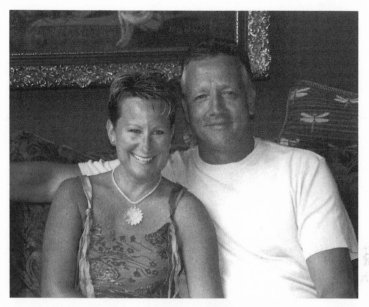

Summer 2003. After a lot of hard days. Although I continued to worry about the cancer returning, happier days had arrived!

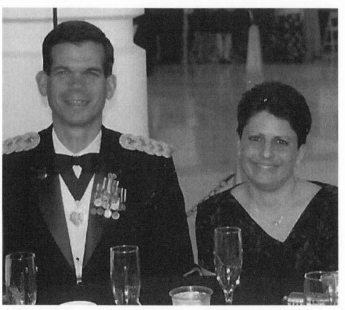

June 2003. Colonel and Mrs. Craig Shriver. We met them at the wedding of Katie Harman and Tim Ebner in Portland, Oregon. Thank you Colonel Shriver for your help with this book!

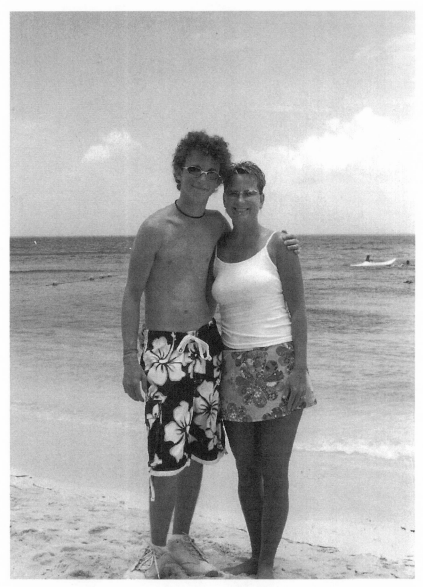

Summer 2003. With my sweet Colby at Moon Palace in Cancun, Mexico! I loved any time we got to spend together! The fresh air and sunshine are very therapeutic and healing for me!

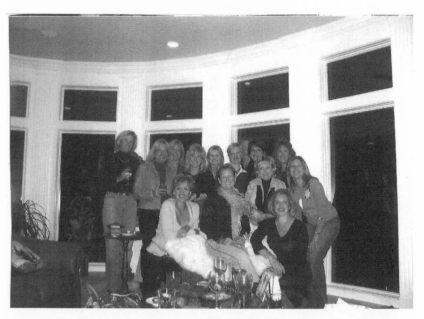

My surprise 40th birthday party! Who said I would never see 40? A girl can never have too many friends! I have been blessed!

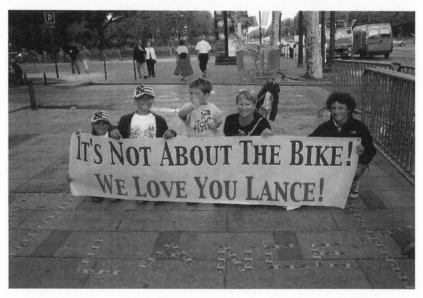

Paris, July 2004. Grand Finale of the Tour de France – Lance Armstrong remains one of my heroes!

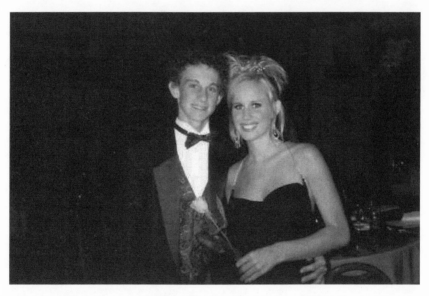

October 2004. Meet me in Paris! Our first double date with Colby and Kenzie at the Touched By Cancer Foundation Gala.

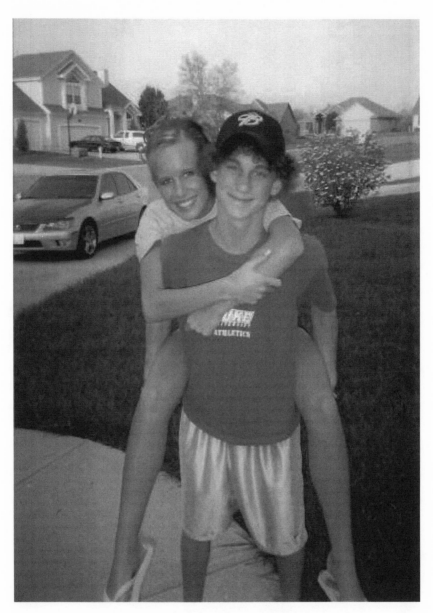

Kenzie and Colby. I am so glad he experienced young love!

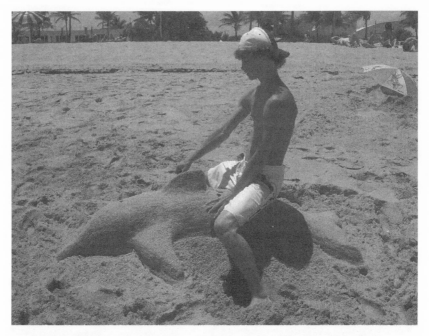

Fort Lauderdale Beach. My last Mother's Day with Colby and Kenzie …

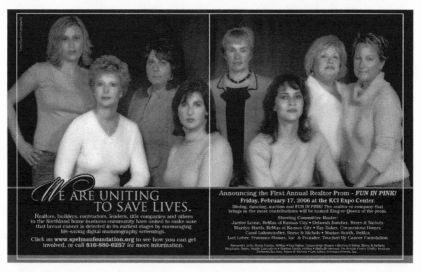

I was able to give Colby a sneak peak before this was published…he was so proud of how well I was doing with my cancer journey! (Tracy Routh Photography)

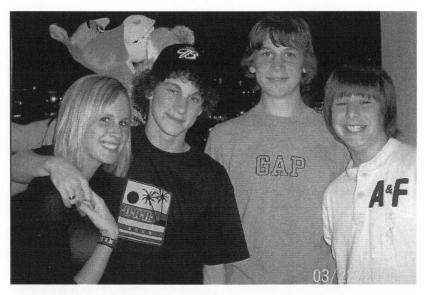

Kenzie, Colby, Anthony, Danny. Times like this will be cherished forever!

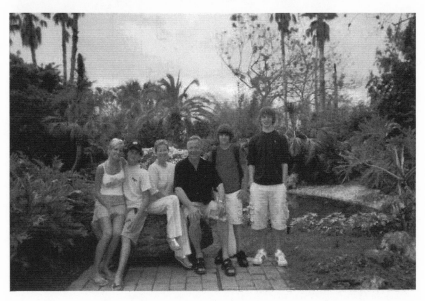

Spring 2005 . Orlando, Florida -- All of us together!

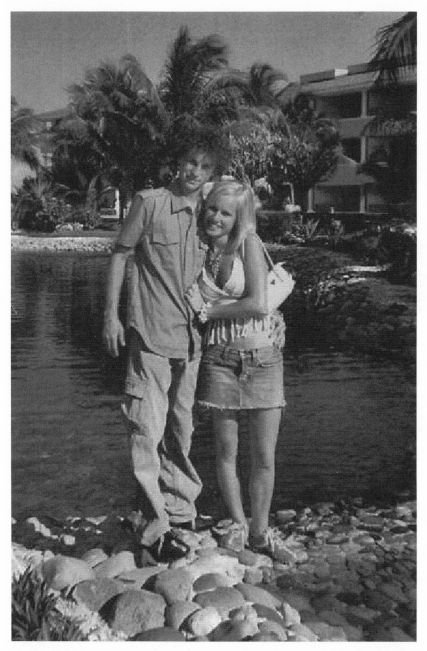

Snuck a quick trip to Moon Palace in Cancun with Kenzie and Colby between his session at the UMKC School of Medicine and the fall semester at UMKC.

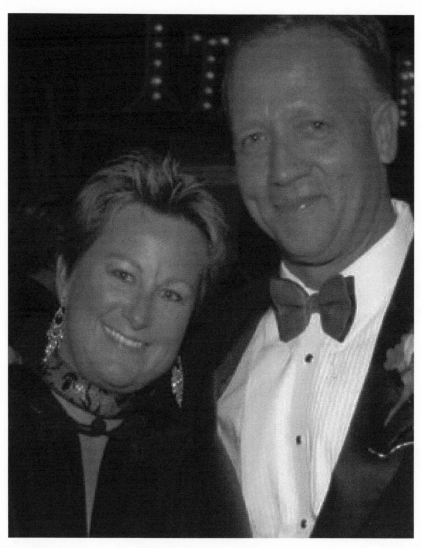

2005 Touched By Cancer Gala.

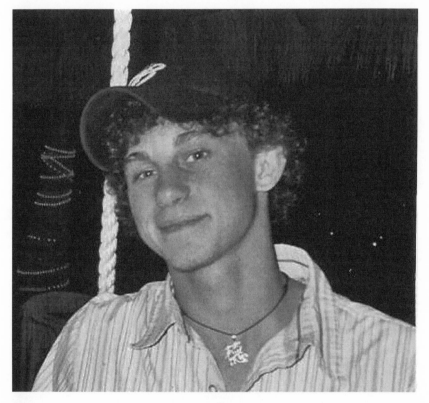

Colby

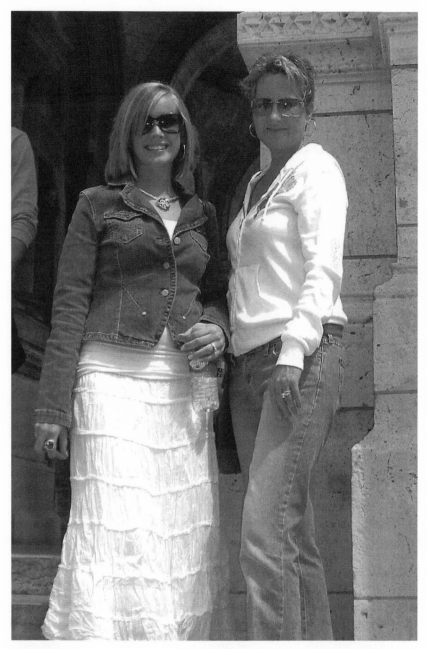

With Kenzie in Paris for her 18th birthday - we shed tears missing Colby but loved our week there ...

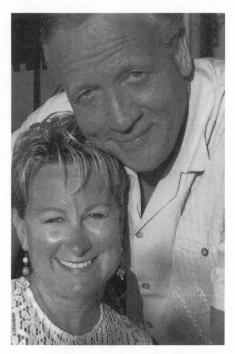

September 2006. We celebrated another milestone by renewing our wedding vows on our 10th Anniversary! We enjoyed the trip to Costa Rica with John and Jami Hepting!

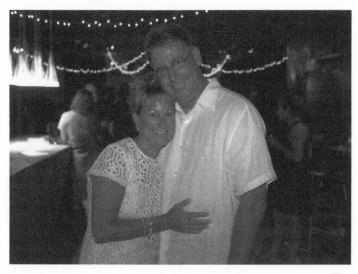

My brother Larry. He has endured so much! Together we've been strong! Love you Larry!

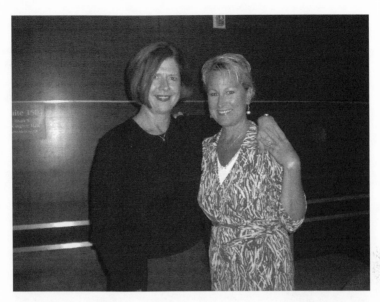

My first public book signing at Menorah Medical Center's Breast Cancer Awareness Event in 2006. Here I am with the publisher of Kansas City Magazine, Katie van Luchene.

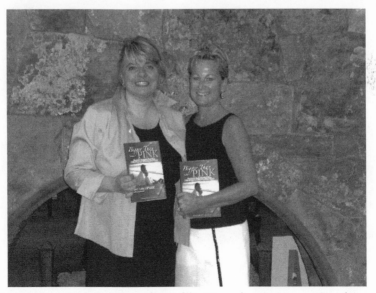

Meeting Geri Higgins, owner of Portfolio Home here in Kansas City, has truly been a gift.

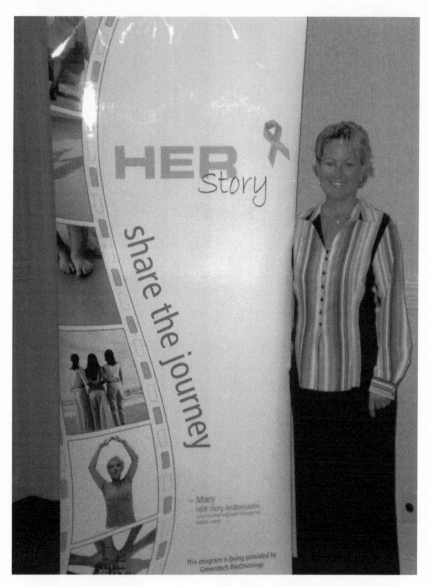

Becoming a HerStory ambassador for Genentech was a great honor.

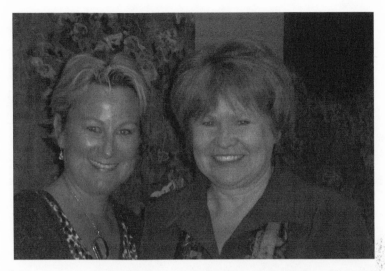

While in St Louis, I also caught up with Bev Vote, the publisher of Breast Cancer Wellness Magazine and a dear friend!

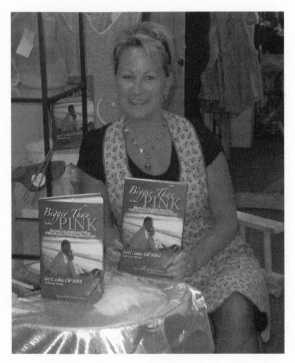

Bigger Than Pink book signing at Eclectics.

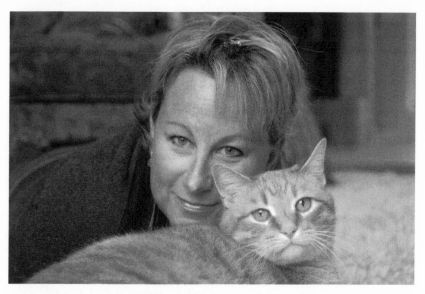

Fuzzy Photos, spring of 2007. Cosmo is my healing cat - faithfully by my side for the whole journey! (Photo by Elaina Generally Photography)

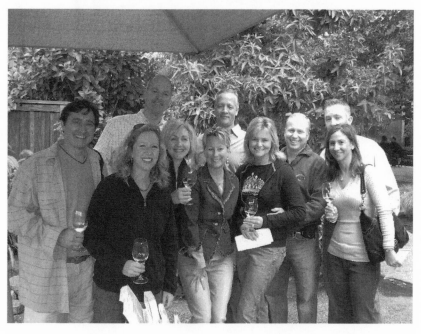

Fabulous wine-tasting trip in Napa with our friends.

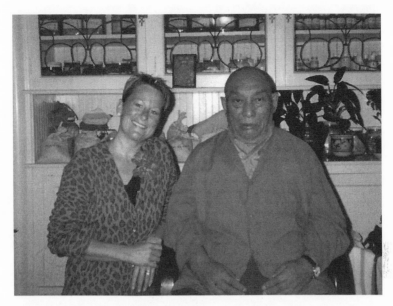

I started seeing Dr. Yeshi Dhonden October, 2001. I continue to see him every year during his U.S. visits! He gives me strength and courage to fight for my life. Truly an angel on Earth!

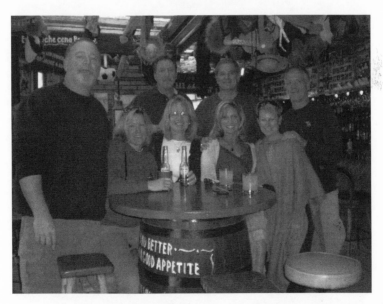

Rosarita Beach, Mexico. Celebrating the memory of Colby one year after, it felt good to laugh and cry with my friends

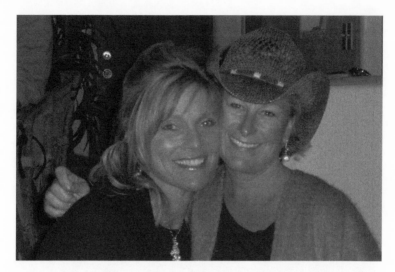

My friend Rozanne Scimeca. I wonder what I would have done without Rozanne and Phil in that year.

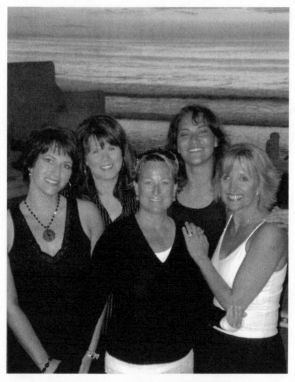

My best friends gathered with me at Rosarita Beach…ending a bittersweet week.

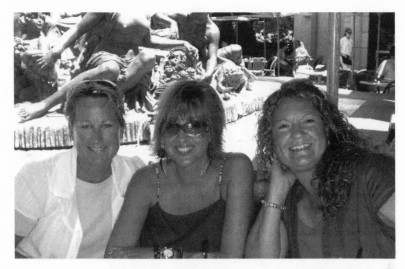

Laura and me with Angie Prindle - brainstorming about bringing the story of my cancer journey to life as a children's book…Princess Elle. Thank you Laura!

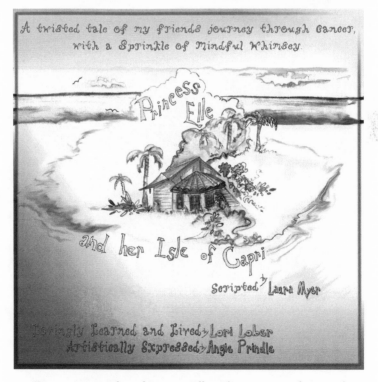

Front cover graphic of Princess Elle. This is going to be so cool!

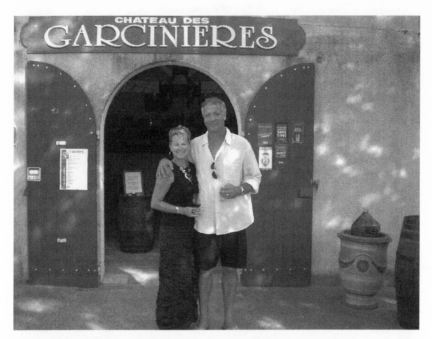

Celebrating our 10th anniversary wine tasting in the south of France, so romantic!

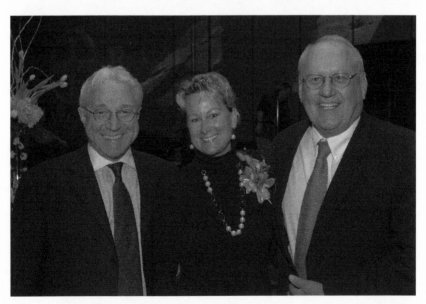

*Kansas City Life Sciences event with President and CEO of Biotech- Jim Green-
wood and President of Kansas City Life Sciences - Bill Duncan.*

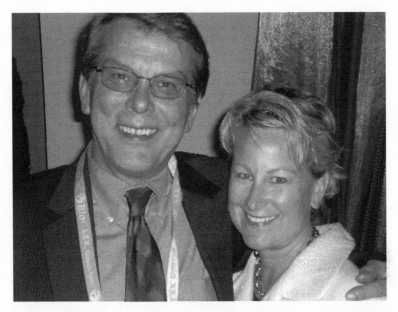

Mr. David Welch sent me a video of Colby taken by Biotech in the spring before we lost him…it is the last video of Colby – something I will treasure always. Thank you David!

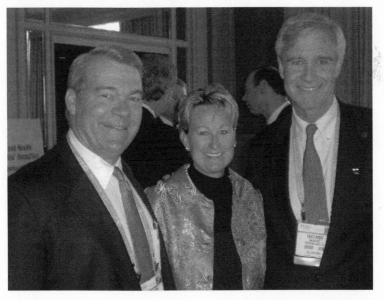

The gentlemen standing with me were instrumental in the development of Herceptin! What an honor to be able to thank them in person!

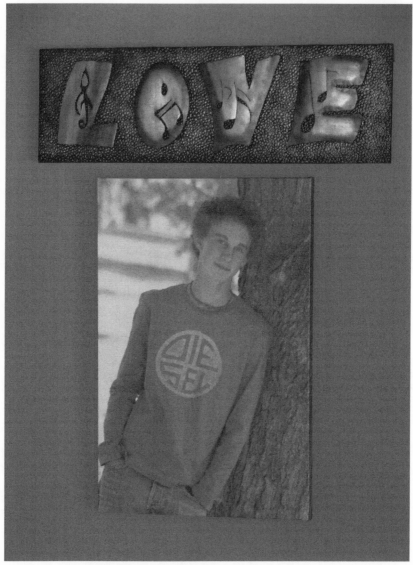

The dedication of the Colby Pavilion 070707

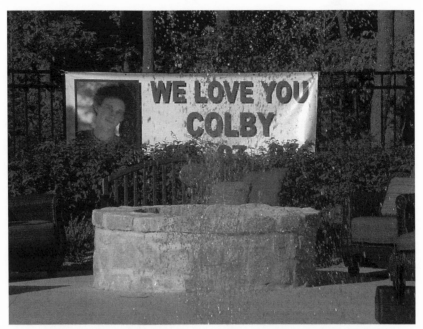

Colby pavilion and banner! 070707—Celebration of Colby's life!

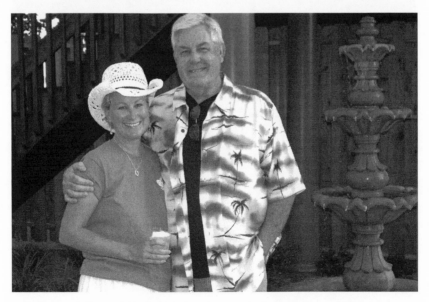

With my dad. He's endured so much through the years too.

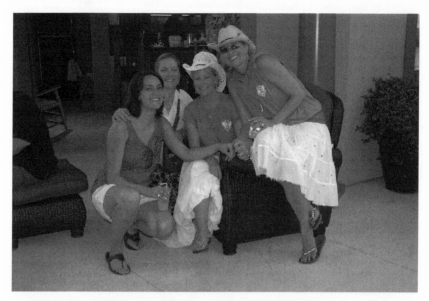

With my friends Michelle, Karen, and Laura.

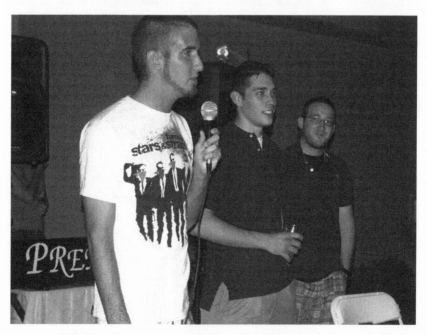

Three best friends remembering Colby. Mike, Chris and Matt!

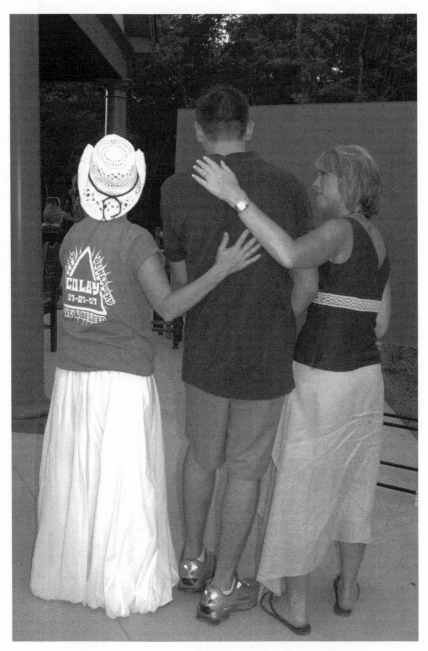

We all support each other, even after a year had passed.

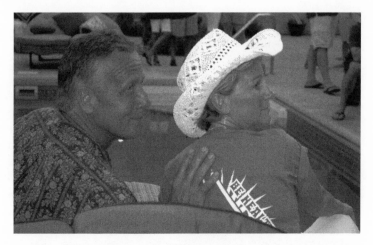

A touching moment as the balloons are released to the heavens.

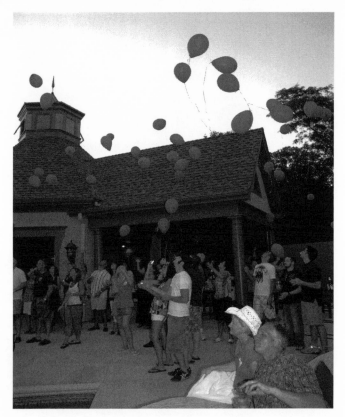

Loving memories take flight.

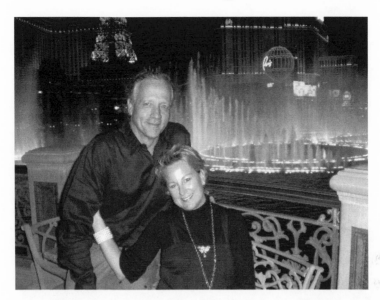

Our trip to Las Vegas fulfilling our promise to Colby -- a trip to Vegas on his 21st birthday.

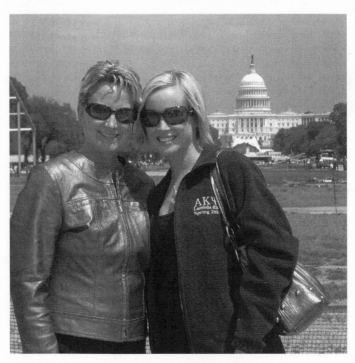

Lori goes to Washington!

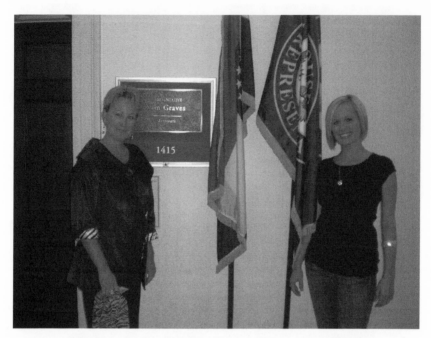

Washington D.C. Outside of our US Congressman's office.

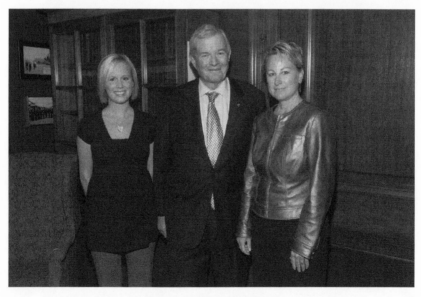

Kenzie and me with our US Senator Kit Bond. We were in Washington to speak on behalf of the Biotech Industry.

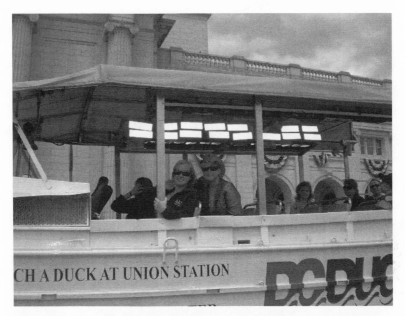

DC Ducks, what a "quack up!" We continue to live life to the fullest!

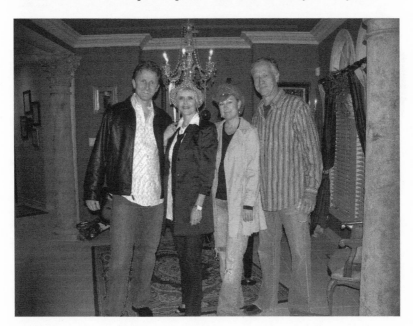

Niek and Vicki Lagerwey, fellow HerStory Ambassadors and great friends flew in from North Carolina to go with us to see Nickelback and Daughtry in concert.

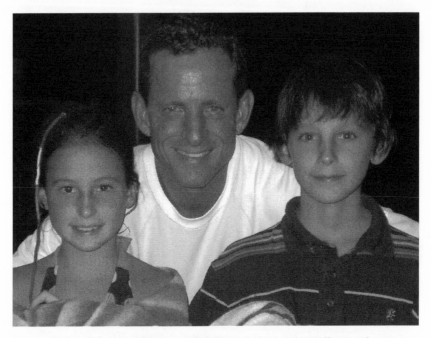

Colby's dad, Jim McLain with Seth and Alex at the Colby Pavilion.

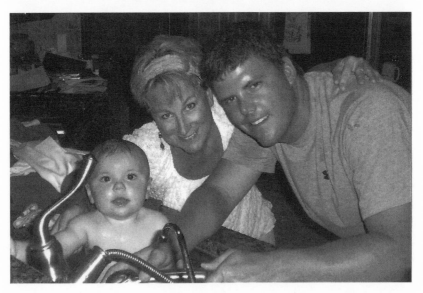

With our cousin Willie and his son Drake! Life is good!

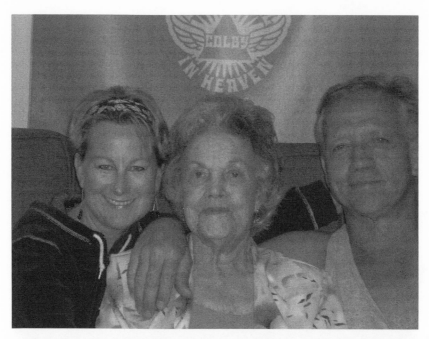

With John's mom Helen. She turns 92 in 2009 – and LOVES her IsAgenix!

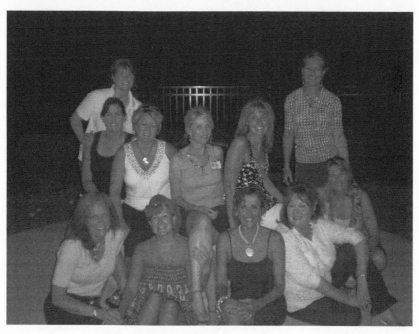

Summer 2008. The Power of 10 - women supporting women!

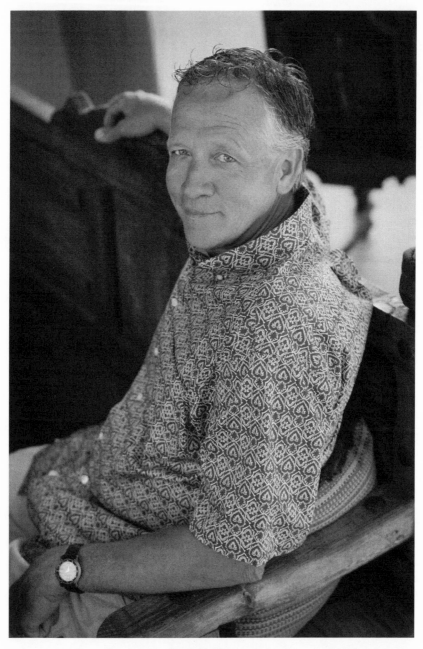

John – the new face for Ralph Lauren? (In my eyes, he is!)

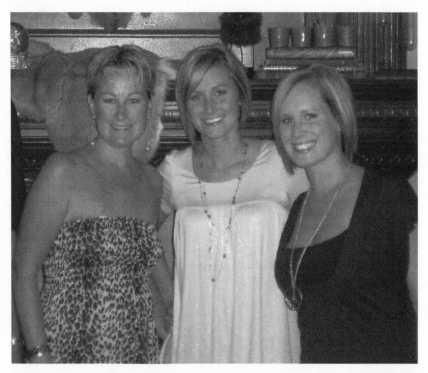

Summer 2008. My 6° of separation from American Idol David Cook: Chelse was David Cook's senior prom date at Blue Springs South! Kenzie, Chelse, and me before the American Idol concert in Kansas City. (And, I had been on IsAgenix for 6 months at the time this photo was snapped!)

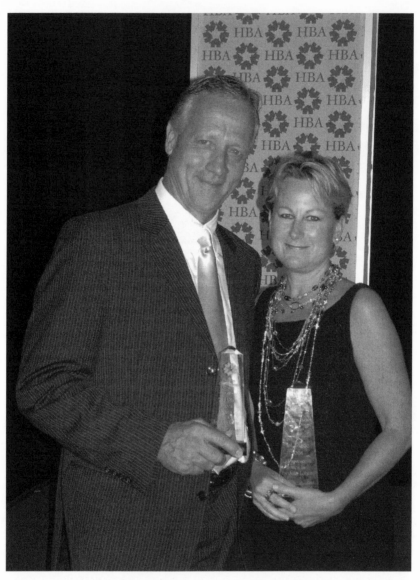

We were thrilled when Provence Homes garnered the 2008 Distinctive Plan and Design Contest Award-sponsored by the Home Builders Association of Greater Kansas City. Another great year!

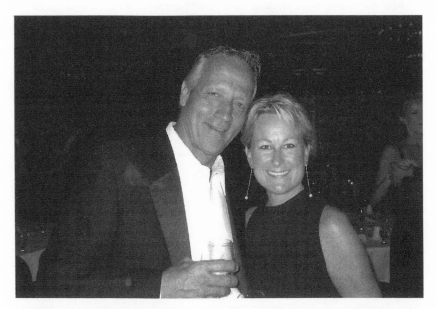

At the 2008 Touched By Cancer Foundation Kaleidoscope of Hope Gala.

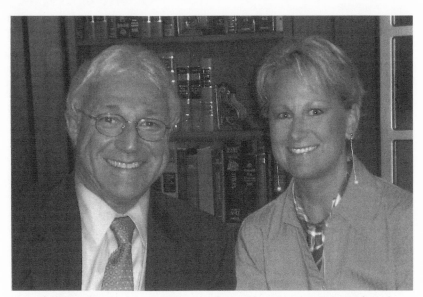

Last fall I participated in a satellite media tour to create awareness about how the biotechnology industry is fighting cancer. I am honored to be working with the Honorable Jim Greenwood, the president and CEO of Biotech.

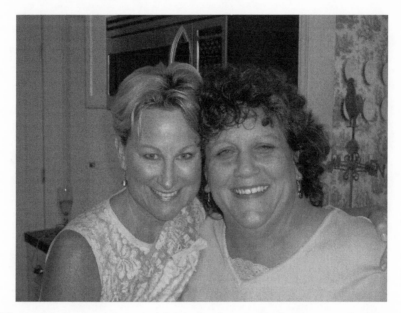

The reason Katie and I connected: Her lovely mom Darla Harman who believed in me and has supported me and my cancer journey since day one.

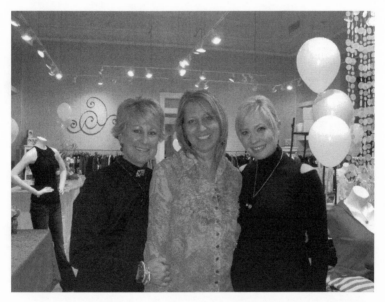

October 2008. With Katie and Julie Lushbaugh at one of the events Katie and her sweet friends put together in Klamath Falls to raise funds and awareness for the Touched By Cancer Foundation.

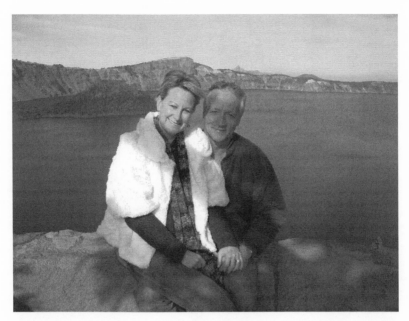

With John at Crater Lake. The pose is reminiscent of our last trip to Colorado with Colby so long ago.

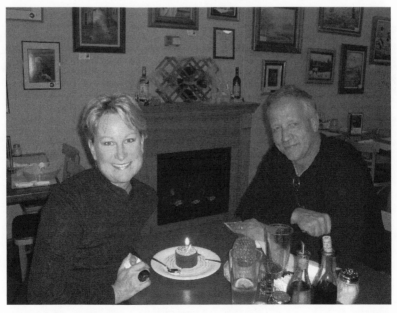

My birthday 2008. Celebrating while visiting Katie, Tim and Tyler in Klamath Falls, Oregon.

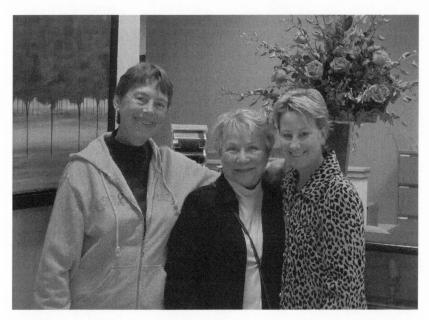

With two of my Earth Angels, Sandy and Judy. Always ready to help at the Touched By Cancer Foundation Wellness Center! Their smiles mean so much! I love you both!

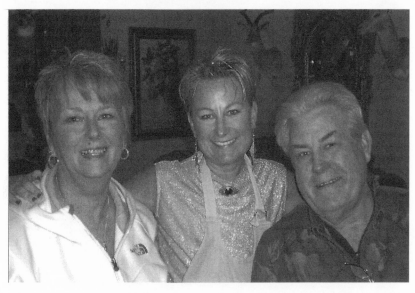

Christmas Day 2008. With my parents Sheila and Larry Wittmeyer. Together, we're hanging in there following the blows we've taken.

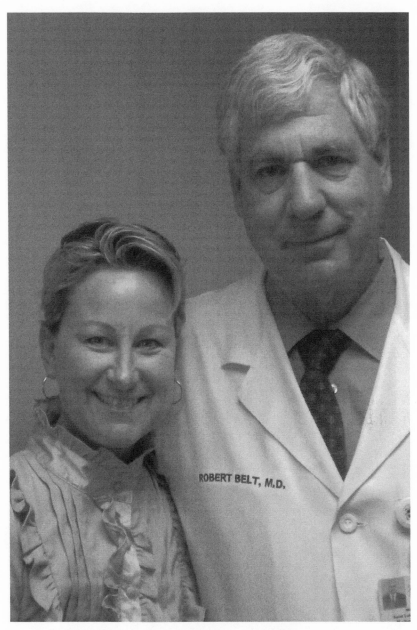

Me & my KC Oncologist, Dr. Robert Belt. It's been great having him on my team back to optimal health and wellness.

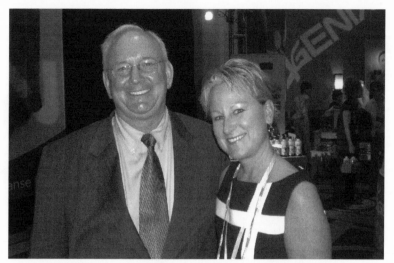

With Dr. Bill Wheeler - ISAGENIX CHIEF SCIENCE OFFICER. He served as MD for two U. S. Presidents! Is that cool; or what?!

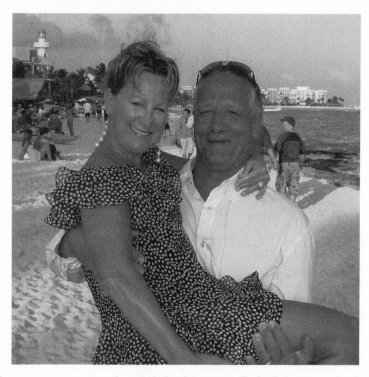

John continues to carry me through the hard times! I really think I'm going to be ok now!

Chapter 6

The Power of Colonics

"An unhealthy colon is toxic to the body and cancer feeds off impurities. You can either allow your colon to be a means for cancer to become stronger and possibly metastasize, or you can empower the colon to produce an environment that is in effect "too healthy and efficient" for cancer to prevail."

As you may guess, a colonic has to do with the colon. The small intestine and the colon – the large intestine – are the body's vessels for transporting bodily waste from the stomach to the rectum. There are other organs and glands that assist in this process and they are directly impacted by the condition of the colon; but make no mistake about it, the colon can affect every aspect of the body, either directly or indirectly. Our body's organ systems are designed to work together in concert so what affects a given organ, will likely affect others. An unhealthy colon is toxic to the body and cancer feeds off impurities. You can either allow your colon to be a means for cancer to become stronger and possibly metastasize, or you can empower the colon to produce an environment that is in effect "too healthy and efficient" for cancer to prevail.

While cancer may thrive on our weaknesses, the body feeds off its own strengths. By strengthening the colon you can also improve the kidneys, the liver, the heart, the mind, the immune system, and so on.

Under normal circumstances the body is well equipped to neutralize and dispose of toxins through the liver, spleen, and other eliminative channels. However, as a stage IV cancer patient, my circumstances were far from "normal". I felt I needed to do more to augment my conventional medicine treatment plan, to help increase my chances of survival.

Colonics is another complementary therapy I chose to employ. I feel colonics positively impacted the results of my conventional treatment. While certainly not obvious, the colon needs to be cared for in order to achieve wellness. The colon affects the overall functions of the body and so its empowerment is essential. The food you eat is processed through the body in a way that aims to make full use of all nutrients to produce energy that is needed in order for the body to function properly. These nutrients are transported throughout the entire body, from glands to organs, from organs to organ systems. The colon is one of the main processes of this transportation. If it is not functioning properly, the body and all of its components will not receive the proper level of nutrients needed.

The colon transfers waste from the food we eat to the rectum where it is expelled from the body. As a result of improper nutrition and environmental toxins, the colon can become clogged with putrefied waste which disrupts the process of elimination and leads to more putrefaction. Maintaining proper digestive and eliminative functions entails having two to three bowel movements per day on a regular basis. Most people are not aware of this. Infants offer a good illustration: ask any mother – a baby will eat and almost immediately eliminate. Their new digestive systems have not had time to develop the mal-absorption problems caused by improper diet, environmental toxins and stress. Faulty digestion and elimination develop in an individual through years of improper lifestyle and dietary habits.

Proper Nutrition. There is much that you can do to improve the condition and functioning of your colon by eating the proper foods. Proper nutrition is lacking in our society. The overall diet of the population in the United States consists mainly of high sodium, sugar, red meat, and processed foods that contribute to the putrefaction that occurs in the colon. Much of the fatty acids and toxic chemicals that are in red meats and processed foods for example, are collected along the walls of the colon in putrefied fecal matter. While the body does manage to absorb what nutrients it can from these foods, they produce a greater proportion of matter that is unnecessary and even harmful. These foods do not help to cleanse, but rather, their by-products collect and become toxic to the body. The overall result is an over-abundance of waste and a lack of nutrition.

Before I was diagnosed with cancer, like most Americans, I enjoyed fast foods like buffalo chicken wings, cheeseburgers, etc. Having a fresh, green salad or some steamed vegetables every now and then was definitely not enough. My cancer diagnosis required that I eat foods that could strengthen my body, help fight the cancer and increase my chance of long-term survival. I needed foods that contained an abundance of nutrients that my body could use to empower itself. The nutrient that best serves the colon is fiber.

Fiber exists in foods such as beans, seeds, raw fruits, and vegetables. These foods also contain the vitamins and minerals that the body needs to function at its best without producing a large amount of excess waste. Many people refer to fruits and vegetables as roughage and this interpretation is accurate in that their rough texture often serves to sweep through the colon, collecting some of the putrefied waste that exists along its walls. When you eat such foods and your bowel movements seem to increase, it is not because more waste has been produced, but because in addition to a normal amount of waste, these fiber-rich foods are carrying along what had already existed and putrefied in the colon.

Colon Irrigation. As discussed earlier, putrefaction is basically the collection of waste around the inner walls of the colon, which directly interferes with the absorption of nutrients and the elimination of needless waste. In my opinion, the best way to keep this from occurring is the process of colon irrigation. While these two words may conjure some unpleasant thoughts, I anticipate that this chapter will convey the message that the benefits of the procedure outweigh its unpleasantness. For me, the benefits of colonics, including colon irrigation, produced comforting results that proved effective. I actually felt so good following a colon therapy session I felt I could do cartwheels out to the car!

Eating the right foods is only part of what is needed to ensure a healthy colon. While it may seem that proper nutrition is a reasonable solution, in my opinion, colon irrigations are still a necessity. Chances are that you have not eaten properly on a consistent basis throughout your life and quite possibly for your entire life. This being so, the amount of putrefaction that has continually accumulated up to now, must be taken into account.

The consumption of proper foods can only cleanse your colon in the length of time it takes for them to pass through your system. Your colon may require greater focus and care to achieve a thorough cleansing (especially if you are over thirty). In many cases, the colon becomes so clogged that even the most beneficial foods cannot entirely pass through the colon. Food could collect and then putrefy along the colon's walls. In this event, your body actually becomes unable to absorb all of the nutrients you consume. This alone, greatly weakens your body's ability to function properly and can be very detrimental to your health and wellness. Fortunately, colonics is a worthwhile solution to this problem.

In the book entitled *Colon Health: The Key to a Vibrant Life*, Dr. Norman W. Walker states, "one should receive at least six colon irrigations every year" in order to ensure a healthy colon. While you should receive a number of irrigations annually, do not be deterred, for it is not an exhausting process. Colon irrigations are not grueling, painful treatments. Irrigations cleanse and massage the interior of the colon by releasing small increments of water into the colon throughout a time period of thirty to forty-five minutes. While it may be awkward to have another individual perform this treatment on you, it is not painful (just remind yourself why you are having it done). You will gradually become more comfortable with the process once you experience the positive results that follow. What can be accomplished in a relatively short time period is well worth the effort it takes to find a qualified colonics practitioner (a Certified Colon therapist) and receive the treatment. In doing so, your body will become able to absorb all nutrients and process all waste without complications. This will energize your body and allow it to fight your illness by surrounding and attacking the plaguing invasion on a healthy front.

Colon irrigations also increase wellness by detoxifying the body. Red meats and processed foods contain toxins that collect and putrefy in the colon. Once consumed, these toxins are released into the body. Once they accumulate in putrefied waste, their toxicity increases. If you leave a glass of water out on a table for a few days, it will become contaminated. If the water was impure when it was first poured, then its quality will become even more unsanitary. While water does not contain its own filtration system, fortunately, our bodies do. Even so, eventual maintenance is required given that this system was not meant to prevail over an imbalance of abundant waste and limited nutrients (there is only so much we can expect of our bodies!).

Over time, the developed mass of rancid waste ferments and the colon becomes increasingly more polluted. As your body continues to carry out its filtration process, some of the toxins that have fermented in your colon are absorbed in the mix of incoming nutrients and passed through your blood to other organs and organ systems. This is why you must continually guard against putrefaction and fermentation.

A synonym of the word 'ferment' is 'turmoil', which is exactly what cancer creates within your body. An antonym for turmoil is order, such as the organized functioning of a clean and healthy colon. This effect can be achieved through colon irrigations and proper nutrition. In other words, order is the solution to chaos and one of the keys to eliminating cancer.

If you truly want to not only survive but to thrive, seek out all treatment options that create stability, evaluate the feasibility of each for your own unique situation, and seize those opportunities which offer the greatest promise. Colonics is an option that I believe put me in a much stronger position to fight off cancer.

We have discussed how colonics allows your body to properly absorb nutrients, and how it detoxifies your body by preventing the fermentation of putrefied waste. However, there is yet another potential benefit colonics can provide.

Putrefaction causes abnormal inflammation or swelling of the colon and can cause physical pressure upon organs that are in close proximity to an inflamed colon. This inflammation can also affect the liver, kidneys, pancreas, spleen, reproductive organs, diaphragm, and stomach.

The choices you make and the actions you take will dictate the wellness of your body. Choosing colonics could be a big step forward in your road to recovery. I challenge you to seriously consider this option and its many benefits. You can cleanse your body of toxins and prevent the harm they cause. Your body will absorb nutrients and produce an abundance of energy that is ever-flowing in the right direction.

In converting your illness into wellness, you learn to strengthen your mind and body so that its systems interact with each other in a way which promotes the proper functioning of a healthy, fit body. You must continue to have a positive and active attitude. Seek out a certified colon therapist in your area and see for yourself how cleansed you feel afterward. Remember, you want to be constantly moving forward toward your long-term survival. I believe colonics is a key factor that will greatly assist you in doing so. The power that you have is limitless. Use it and you will prevail.

NOTE: Colon cleansing or colonics should not be confused with the nutritional and cellular cleansing with the IsAgenix product line. Again, I am not a doctor and the information in this book is provided for educational and informational purposes only. I am simply sharing my experience and incorporating another complementary modality into my wellness regimen. We are not attempting to prescribe, treat, or recommend and in no way is the information contained in this book intended to be a substitute for a health care provider's consultation. If you are ill please consult your own physician or appropriate health care provider.

Chapter 7

The Power of Body Work

"Body Work doesn't just feel good. Research shows it reduces the heart rate, increases the blood circulation and lymph flow, relaxes muscles, improves range of motion, increases endorphins (the body's natural pain killers) and more."

It was May 1, 2000 and I had just received my first chemotherapy treatment at the M.D. Anderson Cancer Center (MDACC) in Houston, Texas. The same evening, we were to attend an awards banquet immediately following our flight to Kansas City from Houston. The banquet was the local Home Builder Association's "American Dream Award" ceremony. My husband John, son Colby and I attended the event. I felt like all my home-building industry colleagues, friends and acquaintances looked at me differently that evening – "Now I am different – I have cancer" is how I felt. Some offered genuine sympathy, while others seemed afraid of me – as if they were afraid they may "catch cancer" from me. It was a very strange night. Nine years later, I still remember telling myself that night, "This is NOT the end of Lori Lober." I was convinced that the clinical trial I was participating in at MDACC was a great choice, but in my heart and soul I continued to feel that I needed to do more.

I'm not sure why, but the first thing I did after we returned home from Houston was visit a book store near our home in Kansas City. For some reason, I couldn't wait to research reflexology, to explore any possible contribution it may make to my overall wellness. I had no prior knowledge of reflexology. What I did know about it was that each point in the hands and feet is somehow related to specific points in the body. It was time for me to get serious. Once again, I needed to take matters into my own hands and further coordinate my "journey to wellness".

I purchased several books on reflexology that day. I looked at the diagrams and focused on the points representing key areas of my body — my breasts, my liver, my lymphatic system, etc. Because cancer had spread throughout my lymphatic system, I felt I should research that as well. I immediately began to treat myself. Every now and then, my husband John would do it for me. I visualized all the cancer leaving my body as I would treat myself, sometimes so vigorously that my fingers would hurt from the pressure I was applying. Each day I would give myself these "treatments", sometimes as often as three times a day! It would be a little while however, before I sought professional treatment, as life was about to offer me one of its more pleasant unexpected surprises.

My Forever Friend. I had been continuously putting the word out that I was very eager to find another stage IV breast cancer patient who was doing well. I knew she was out there and if I could find her, she would give me hope! One day John called me — he had just spoken with one of our Provence homeowners who had heard of my recent cancer diagnosis. She believed that one of her neighbors had exactly the same type of cancer I had and she was doing exceptionally well! Without skipping a beat, I picked up the phone and called our client to discuss this with her.

Within a few days, Connie and I talked on the phone. We compared stories. It was so incredibly comforting to speak with someone who understood everything I was feeling. She knew the lingo, she could relate to my fears – she was my angel on earth! I was so happy. She was cute and spunky and she was *beating the odds*!

After meeting Connie and witnessing her strength, I never again felt sorry for myself. She inspired me to fight like hell and now I knew that I, too, could truly win --- I could beat cancer and she was proof!

Connie and I would have lunch together and talk about our husbands and our kids. We would talk about proper nutrition and what she was juicing as we chatted on the phone first thing in the morning. We would talk about anything and everything that was currently consuming our lives. Of course 99% of it revolved around our cancer journey. We became fast and close friends.

I told Connie of my desire to begin receiving therapeutic massage and professional reflexology. She had a wonderful friend that did therapeutic massage! If Connie believed in her and trusted her, that was enough for me. I first met Vonnie, a retired nurse who had practiced therapeutic massage for 16 years, just two months into my "journey to wellness". Not only did I feel it was important to professionally treat my lymphatic system with massage, but it could help alleviate stress as well. Living each day with the realization that I may be dying, was and still is extremely stressful. While there is currently "no evidence of disease" in my body, the knowledge that the cancer can return can, at times, be stressful and draining. It is key for cancer patients to control and limit stress in their daily lives because cancer cells can "feed" off stress. Additionally, the side effects of two rounds of chemotherapy were beginning to slow me down.

Therapeutic Massage. Therapeutic massage involves the manipulation of the soft tissue structures of the body. Its goal is to alleviate pain, discomfort, muscle spasms, and stress. The American Massage Therapy Association (AMTA) defines massage therapy as a profession in which the practitioner applies manual pressure with the intention of positively affecting the health and well being of the client. The AMTA works to establish massage therapy as integral to the maintenance of good health and complementary to other therapeutic processes.

I began weekly massage treatments. Vonnie saw me through the first five years and now Jennifer provides these healing sessions in my home. My therapists over the years have been so sweet — one even offered a discounted price to cancer patients! I have regarded my hour-long therapeutic massage sessions as wellness appointments and with only one or two exceptions, have never missed my appointments. Boy, in the last nine years, have my massage therapists seen me at my worst!

Massage does more than feel good. In my opinion, for anyone fighting cancer it's not a luxury; it's a necessity! Research shows it reduces the heart rate, increases the blood circulation and lymph flow, relaxes muscles, improves range of motion, increases endorphins (the body's natural pain killers) and more. This was especially beneficial after my double-mastectomy. Therapeutic massage definitely helps me feel less anxious and stressed. A writer for the "*Chicago Tribune*" stated, "Massage is to the human body what a tune-up is to an automobile." I will continue to receive therapeutic massage as part of my ongoing wellness program!

Reflexology. Reflexology is a science that deals with the principle that there are reflexes in the feet and hands relative to each and every organ in the body. By properly working on these reflexes, reflexology can help to relieve many health problems in a natural way. Some form of reflexology was practiced by the Egyptians as early as 2330 BC. Reflexology as we know it was first researched and developed in America during the 1930's and 1940's. Today, there are thousands of reflexologists practicing all over the world.

In my opinion, the best way to find a qualified and respected therapist is by personal referral. I was fortunate that Vonnie was able to point me in the direction of a wonderful reflexologist. I had continued to do reflexology on myself until I found Paula! Paula was more than a reflexologist to me. She became a wonderful friend! We visited the entire appointment. We shared healthy recipes. We dished on husbands and kids and friends, and most importantly, we prayed together. Like therapeutic massage, I had a standing wellness appointment with Paula every week. Unless the weather was horrific,

I showed up without fail. It takes a dedication to wellness to keep all the various weekly appointments, but I knew I could never "fall off the wagon", back into my old routine. After all, my previous lifestyle choices could very likely have played a role in my cancer in the first place, right?

In July 2002, John, Colby and I went to Africa to celebrate John's 45th birthday. What a gift that trip was! Because of the extended travel time to our destination, I asked the safari camp to please locate a reflexologist so the three of us could receive a treatment. They found a reflexologist who agreed to drive two hours each way to come to our camp and give us reflexology and therapeutic massage treatments! This would be John's first reflexology treatment, and as it turned out, was very timely.

During his treatment the reflexologist found an enlarged adrenal gland and John said it was sore to the touch. She explained this was most likely due to a high level of stress. She worked the area, but suggested John get a reflexology treatment when we arrived back in the States. A week or so later, John began receiving treatments from my reflexologist, Paula. She too, felt the same spot and concurred that John's level of stress was very high and advised him to have a series of treatments. Gradually, the enlarged spot on his foot went away. Who knows what John may have experienced without the healing provided by reflexology? Today John swears by reflexology! Currently John and I both continue regular reflexology treatments with Karen Kipp. She not only provides great healing treatments in our home, she was instrumental in the opening of the Touched By Cancer Wellness Center. Thank you Karen!

Reflexology is something I highly recommend for cancer patients as it can also help normalize the body's functions and promote natural healing. It treats the entire body, not just specific organs. It promotes integration of mind and emotions, and helps relieve stress. Many common and serious illnesses are directly linked to stress, and relieving it, allows the body to heal itself naturally.

As a cancer patient, I believe in chemotherapy and surgery (as long as surgery is performed at the proper time as determined by a multi-disciplinary team of physicians, not the surgeon alone). I also know that long-term survival rates do not seem to be improving when patients adhere solely to Western medicine. Incorporating non-invasive, drug-free treatments like therapeutic massage and reflexology that provide effective results seems like a no-brainer to me. Incorporating everything possible to increase my odds of long-term survival has become my way of life and in spite of everything I have been through, I have never felt better. I believe reflexology and therapeutic massage have played a key role in my journey to wellness!

As with any complementary or alternative treatment, please consult your physician(s) prior to beginning body work if you have been diagnosed with cancer, especially lymphoma. I was advised by my physician to discontinue yoga when an inexplicable "hot spot" or an area of increased activity/blood flow was detected on a PET scan several years ago. I am honored and proud to say that my oncologist reported to me on January 2, 2009 that even this hot spot has decreased in size and can barely be seen now!

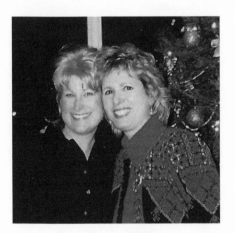

Connie & Lori
December, 2000 – My memory of Connie will never fade.
She passed to a better place in October 2002, instilling
within me a never-ending strength to fight like hell!

Connie's cancer returned, and after a long, valiantly fought battle, she passed away in October 2002. Sometimes, even if we do everything in our power — everything "right", we are unable to overcome this horrible disease. Connie is an angel, only now in Heaven, and her spirit continues to guide me, even today. Every time I see a feather, I think of her and my Sweet Colby!

Chapter 8

The Power of Chiropractic Care!

"Now what?" ... after the chemo, and the chiropractic and the surgery and the vitamins and minerals and herbs, what do YOU do to create a pure and sufficient body where cancer does not grow.

Bruce Rippee, D.C., C.C.W.P.

Throughout my cancer journey I had visited a chiropractor on and off. Even though I totally understand the importance of keeping the inner structure of our bodies healthy and aligned for optimal performance, chiropractic care was not something I included in my regular wellness routine before the cancer. Looking back, regular chiropractic care could have supported my heavily taxed body in fighting the breast cancer throughout my lymphatic system and distant metastasis in my liver. And as I go forward in my evolving wellness journey, recent personal experience and those of close friends led me back to chiropractic care and it is now a regular part of my self-care and overall health and wellness routine.

Recently, I became a re-dedicated, loyal and committed fan of chiropractic care. In early 2008, I was in Paris, France on spring break with Kenzie, her sister Chelse and my dear friend Cheryl

Lewis. About half way through the week, I found I could not walk! The pain became progressively worse and worse. It was so bad that after the long flight back to the United States, I could not even walk to deplane. I have always prided myself for my high tolerance to pain but this was beyond my pain threshold. I was humiliated having to call for a wheelchair to help me off the plane, get through U. S. Customs and Immigration and onto our connecting flight home. Thank goodness for my dear, sweet travel partners helping with my luggage – for those of you who know me pretty well, you'll vouch that I am not a light traveler!

Needless to say, my husband John was shocked when he pulled up to pick us up at KCI Airport and saw me in a wheelchair. He had to literally carry me into our home. The pain was so severe I had to crawl around the house!

We squeezed into our general M. D. the next morning. After X-Rays and a physical he diagnosed me as having plantar fasciitis. The doctor suggested I see a podiatrist, a foot specialist, for a second opinion. The next day, the podiatrist confirmed the original diagnosis, told me how to exercise my foot and that it could easily be six or seven months of living with this intense pain before it completely healed. My first thought was, "I cannot lay low for six or seven months while this fascia heals – I have too much to do!" To try to make the best of the situation, I purchased the cutest orthotic shoes I could find – STILL NOT SO CUTE!

A Wellness Coach. My husband John happened to be seeing his chiropractor, Dr. Bruce Rippee that day. Even though John had seen Dr. Bruce on and off for the last twelve to thirteen years, I had never met him! What I knew from John and many of our friends is that Dr. Bruce is well-known and loved in Kansas City. During their session, John mentioned my plantar fasciitis and the severe pain I was experiencing. Dr. Bruce asked John to get me on the telephone and thankfully I answered. Dr. Bruce assured me that he could help me and I would NOT have to suffer with this pain for six to seven months!

To my astonishment, in eight to ten appointments with ultrasound and adjustments, I was operating at 70-80%! Each appointment thereafter helped my foot to heal a little bit more. While I was extremely grateful for my healing, I was not sure if this was a fluke. Not until I saw similar results in my dear, dear, sweet friend Phil Scimeca. Phil had been struggling with foot problems for a year or more. He had seen all the specialists, purchased all the orthotics and was even contemplating surgery by this time. I urged Phil and his wife Rozanne to get into see Dr. Bruce before he moved forward with surgery.

After only a few months, Phil and Rozanne were dancing the night away again and walking three plus miles every day! This is another amazing testimonial that affirms my belief in multiple opinions, especially if surgery is the treatment option presented. I will tell you that choosing chiropractic care helped me avoid an unnecessary surgery! Again this is my experience and yours may be very different. I just know that Dr. Bruce has not only been an amazing addition to my wellness team, he is also a fantastic overall health and wellness coach for me and everyone he sees! His philosophy of wellness echoes much of what I have talked about in this book.

Philosophy of Wellness. Well just what is wellness and how does chiropractic care fit into a wellness journey? According to Dr. Bruce Rippee, "Wellness is a philosophy surrounded by hard science that states your body is not genetically predisposed to illness."

Dr. Rippee expands on the state of wellness and how it is achieved:

> "If you can bear with me for a second and see your body as a ecosystem of 70 trillion or so cells, each having a specific job and each needing to replicate itself (so that the new cell can do that job) as a perfect copy of the original. Our bodies reach a state of homeostasis when all of our cells are functioning well and together. Homeostasis is easiest described as the balance that we must attain by removing whatever is

toxic to us and supplying our bodies with whatever it needs. Adaptations in the gene code, such as cancer, are a lack of homeostasis proved by the fact that our genes are designed to produce a healthy, vibrant cell to replace the one that has lived its life. Now would you do me a favor, get online and search for the word, *epigenetics*? I promise that it will give you a measure of hope by basically stating, change the environment for the better and you will change the genetic expression of the organism for the better!

So, why doesn't everyone follow along with cell homeostasis and removing toxicity and deficiency? I was out to brunch with my family on a Sunday and, just like any normal 6 year old girl, my daughter was having trouble grasping the idea of wellness. We had been to church and all of the children in her Sunday school class had a dish of pudding as a snack. Now, although I am never militant about it, she knows very well how I feel about pudding and informs me that she does NOT want a dessert while we are out to brunch because she has already had enough "bad stuff" today. Her eyes widened as she said the word NOT and her voice carried all of the fervor that a little girl can muster. All I said was, "Way to go Lindsey, that is an excellent choice!" Her passionate conviction lasted most of 10 minutes and eventually turned to tears for the simple reason that she knew everyone else was going to have dessert and she wasn't going to be allowed any. She hadn't even seen what was for dessert but the idea of denying herself something that others might have, and she could not, was painful--even if it was toxic.

Isn't this how we all are, really? Everyday I give little tricks to my patients to help them move toward a sufficient and pure environment so that they can heal and live at an optimal level. As I meet every new patient, though, I have learned to first ask them to tell me three things that they are not going to give up no matter how bad it is for them. The most popular answers are, in no particular order: coffee, chocolate, candy, cigarettes (all kinds of tobacco), alcohol (in all varieties,) bread and pasta. This gives me an idea of the rules that I must play by and gives my patients a measure of peace in knowing that I will not force them to change everything all at once. Wellness has to be easy and should always begin with adding something rather than taking something that is perceived as pleasurable away."

How to get started. Jim Wyllie, D.C., DABCO CCWP, suggests that for many of us our first conscious thoughts regarding health come during times of crisis when choices are few, and as a result we resort to available crisis oriented measures to save our life. But what happens once the crisis is averted? Now what? If we do not reset our head we will spend our lives running from the disease we fear (talk about a stress filled lifestyle!) and our mind will create the very disease we fear. This is *epigenetics* (epi = above, genetics = pertaining to genes) at work. Our thoughts control genetic expression and directly influence cell health. Take a few minutes to answer the questions. Think about them. They will help you identify your core beliefs about health and wellness.

- Is it better to stay well, or cycle in and out of pain (problems)?
- Would you rather take supplements to stay well or wait for sickness and take pills?
- Do you innately expect health or disease?
- If you have two people with the same blood pressure reading, but one of them takes medication to lower it, are they equally healthy?
- Did God design you to be healthy or sick?
- Do your choices affect your health?

- If you give your body everything it needs in sufficient quantities, what do you think your chances of being sick and diseased are?
- Can you continually think a negative thought and not have it negatively impact your health?
- Do your genes predestine your health?

Even with a strong personal core belief that every cell of your body is set on health, the odds are astronomically stacked against a successful outcome, if you try to go it alone. You need support. Dr. Rippee and Dr. Wyllie agree you must find a friend, a faithful community, and a wellness coach (i.e., a CCWP) that thinks and believes that as long as there is life there is hope for abundant health.

When choosing a wellness coach to assist in your new wellness lifestyle, look for chiropractors that have a C.C.W.P. after their names. This stands for 'certified chiropractic wellness practitioner' and is a post-doctoral degree from the International Chiropractic Association that means they know how to gently move a person from a toxic and insufficient environment toward a sufficient and pure one. The degree is bestowed upon doctors who complete extensive course work and testing surrounding the scientific research and teachings of James Chestnut.

Dr. Rippee has adapted Dr. Chestnut's six beginning steps emphasizing the incorporation of the wellness philosophy into everyday life:

- **Start by adding sufficiency NOT removing toxicity.** Do not make getting healthy about deprivation. Make it easy and comfortable. Get a wellness coach to give you some fun tricks and movements to try. Please remember that the number one deficiency in America is movement. Adding in fun, gentle movements **EVERY** day is a must to reach homeostasis.

- **Fresh Fiber First. (FFF--easy to remember)** Always eat some raw vegetables or fruit first before **EVERY** snack or meal. It adds antioxidants and phyto-chemicals, vitamins and minerals. It should be a medium apple sized portion at least. My wife stopped eating chocolates in the evening because she knew that in order to follow this rule, she was going to have to eat a bunch of grapes, or an apple, or some kiwi, or an orange...before she should eat the chocolate. When she tried this, she found that the fruit was plenty and that she didn't really need the chocolate anyway.

- **Incorporate activity into your work, family and social lives.** Meet friends for walks or activities rather than food. Incorporate spinal hygiene exercises and some walking into your daily routine. At Chiropractic Life Center here in Kansas City, the entire office closes down from 12-2pm every Monday, Wednesday and Friday so that we can go to the gym and exercise. Everyone goes together and the team building and health and wellness benefits are amazing!

- **Always shop full.** The nutritional decisions that govern your health are made at the point of purchase. If the bad foods don't get purchased, they don't get eaten. No one is going to get up from the couch in the evening, look in the pantry and, not finding double stuffed cookies, go looking for the car keys for a quick run to the store.

- **Always judge your choices based on how you will feel AFTER the choice not before or during.** You will never regret a healthy choice. Evaluate your choices based on what your cells need, not cravings or emotions. How many of us have reached for the double stuffed cookies, ice cream, candy, etc. and 30 minutes later said to ourselves, 'that was SUCH a bad idea!'

- **Begin and end each day with self talk focused on gratitude, optimism and love and forgiveness of self and others.** Evaluate self talk by how it makes you feel. If it doesn't make you feel good, change it. We need to pour love into ourselves, forgive whatever transgressions that yesterday had and use today to further our health. Focus on the positives and keep in that positive moment. You cannot take war out of the world when you hold it in your own heart. Toxic lifestyles are changed by constantly asking ourselves what I can do **TODAY** to further my health and wellness.

Incorporating chiropractic care has become an important part of my wellness journey going forward. The philosophy Dr. Rippee shares fully supports what I have learned over the last nine years. Wellness is an overall lifestyle that you personalize with the choices you make. I urge anyone who is experiencing dis-ease in their body to find the best chiropractor in your area and begin practicing these principles of wellness. I cannot stress enough how my life has changed since I have embraced the many different aspects of wellness!

Chapter 9

The Power of the Biotechnology Industry!

Biological Therapies work with the body's own natural systems to fight cancer and associated side effects. Doctors feel these new therapies are so promising they look to them as one of the top four methods of treatment.

In April, 2000 I can honestly tell you I had no idea what the "Biotechnology Industry" even was or did! Once I was told my cancer had metastasized and progressed to the worst possible stage I was, in my heart and soul, willing to cling to ANYTHING that could offer me HOPE.

My oncologist at M. D. Anderson Cancer Center told me I could be a participant in a clinical trial with a drug called Herceptin. Herceptin is a monoclonal antibody that blocks the oncogene that fed my very aggressive type of pre-menopausal breast cancer. Although neither my oncologist nor Genentech (the manufacturer of this drug) could ever make any promises, this new treatment, when combined with a chemotherapy called Taxotere could offer me HOPE! What was available and approved through the FDA offered me little, if any hope. John and I signed all of the clinical trial paperwork without understanding most of if. We just *BELIEVED* with our hearts and souls we were meant to be at M. D. Anderson

Cancer Center with this team of gifted doctors and we know in our hearts and souls that being part of this clinical trial is one of the reasons I continue to thrive today.

Biological Therapies. Herceptin is a result of the research in the field of biological therapies. Biological therapies work with the body's own natural systems to fight cancer and associated side effects. Doctors feel these new therapies are so promising they look to them as one of the top four methods of treatment. Using these biological tools doctors can detect cancer in earlier stages, target specific cancers, manage side effects, strengthen immune systems, and prolong life. Thanks to the research and development in the biotechnology field, disease in many cases can be managed, or even cured. Some cancers in particular have been found to be susceptible to monoclonal antibodies and other biological therapies. These incredible advances provide hope to those diagnosed with a disease once considered a death sentence.

Here are some things to consider when choosing clinical trials:

- Talk to your doctor about clinical trials you may qualify for. (Take your supporter with you or record the discussion. The information can be overwhelming to take in all at once.)
- What questions should you ask your doctor about clinical trials?(patient care, cost, logistics, potential risks/benefits, personal issues)
- What is informed consent? (understanding the study's approach, risks, interventions, tests, etc.)

The National Cancer Institute has an information-packed section addressing everything you could want to know about participating in a clinical trial. You can research clinical trials and the points above at *www.cancer.gov/CLINICALTRIALS*.

In 2002, my oncologist in Kansas City and I found and researched another clinical trial I could potentially qualify for. John and I were thrilled! Why not? That's when I met Dr. Michael Morse with the Duke Comprehensive Cancer Center and I was accepted as a participant in his dendritic cell immunization study. This was part of the research that led to the discovery of why vaccines in the past have been unsuccessful in treating cancer! And once they know why something will not work, they can move into studying how it can work. Another way biotechnology is being used!

Long story short, I was approached by Genentech and was invited to serve as an ambassador for their "HERSTORY" program. This is something I have always feared – the dreaded public speaking. I am just as nervous in front of groups of ten to twenty. It is not easy for me! My dear friend, Fred Pryor has worked with me. Sweet Katie Harman Ebner has tried – The Honorable James Greenwood, the President and CEO of the Biotechnology Industry is an amazing speaker and he has been a powerful role model - how do they do what they do with such confidence, style and grace? They are **my** idols!

The power of biotechnology continues. In March 2006, I was asked by Kansas City Life Sciences to say a few words at their conference. This would give me the opportunity to thank those whose work was instrumental to my being alive today! Pushing through my fears, I candidly expressed my deep gratitude. To my surprise, I received a standing ovation from the packed house. The Honorable Jim Greenwood, President of the Biotechnology Industry, was the keynote speaker in Kansas City that night. Wowzie! What a brilliant man he is and what an honor to be on the same stage with him!

I continue to tell my story to groups large and small always expressing my feelings of gratitude for the biotechnology industry finding treatments and someday a cure for cancer. As far as overcoming my fear to speak, I garner strength as I see information transform the faces of fear and uncertainty to that of determination and hope. And, I know that Colby gives me the strength along the way!

Chapter 10

The Power of Family & Friends

"When chill winds blow fierce, a friend acts like a torch, guiding you to safety, giving you warmth, comforting you till the storm is over."

Stuart & Linda MacFarlane

Family. What can I say, how much can I say, how can I say it? I will never be able to find the words to show the depth of my love and gratitude for my family's ever-present and unwavering love and support given to me from the day of my diagnosis to this day.

I don't know how I could have survived without the constant support of my husband John. No matter what I wanted to do, what seemingly crazy or unorthodox treatment I proposed trying (that sometimes involved him), he was ok with it. I believe John found his "voice" to speak out against cancer when we found a way to work together for the common cause to fight cancer. Through developing the Touched By Cancer Foundation and the Building Awareness Designer Show Home, he has been able to tap his own expertise and put his many years of experience in the homebuilding industry to use in our joint effort to build awareness and raise funds to fight cancer.

My precious son Colby was only thirteen when I was diagnosed. I continued to drive him the sixty mile roundtrip to and from school daily, even during my most difficult treatments. I enjoyed our car rides and we talked about everything I was going through. He wanted very much to understand what I was experiencing and feeling, and although he was young, he always wanted to know what he could do to help. He listened to me, and at times, he was my pillar of strength. I think he likely grew up faster than his peers. At age 18, his goal was to be a doctor. He witnessed firsthand, the challenges I faced as a cancer patient, and he wanted to be part of the next generation of health care professionals that would understand and recognize the power of combining Western medicine with so-called alternative treatments and complementary modalities. He wanted to give of himself in honor of my journey and our sacrifices as a family, in order to help other families that face terminal illnesses. For me, that gave tremendous meaning to all that I had endured, and offered at least a partial answer to "why did this happen to me?" And now I know that God had another plan for sweet Colby.

Friends. Cancer and friends – for me, both have been a blessing. I realize that to some, it may seem strange to say that cancer has been a blessing — please read on. Just as having and surviving cancer has changed my outlook on life, it has also changed my outlook on friends. Before my diagnosis, I had a wonderful group of friends and after my diagnosis the true friendships blossomed into deeper, more meaningful relationships. Some friendships became strained and psychologically draining and fell apart, never to be repaired. I understand and I believe the whole journey is part of God's plan for me.

Although I have lost friends, the new and deep friendships I have made are real and true. My friends love me for who I am – they're not afraid of me. They're not worried that they can "catch" cancer from me or something crazy like that. (I do think the uninformed still believe that cancer is a communicable disease – in some ways, we have a long way to go!) I do not believe there are any accidents. A friend once told me, "Everyone is in your life for a reason, a season or a lifetime." My experience with cancer has shown me which of my long-time friends are truly there for me, and will continue to be there throughout my lifetime

My Wellness Partner. I want to encourage anyone reading this book to embrace a "Wellness Partner." Over the course of the last six years, my dear friend Laura Myer has been mine. We have traveled to see Dr Yeshi Dhonden together, we go on wellness trips and most importantly, we hold each other accountable! We talk about what we can do to empower our bodies to fight off illness and to operate at optimal health. I have so much gratitude in my heart for her being by my side through thick and thin. After I lost Colby, it was the love and strength of Laura and my dear friend Jami Hepting that carried me through the dark times after that tragic event. I do not know how I would have made it without their loving support. I am eternally grateful to both of them for their friendship.

Family and friends are truly what continues to make my world go 'round! I have been fortunate to travel with them, laugh with them and cry with them. Sharing special anniversaries, holidays, momentous birthdays and events with my family and friends, gives me something wonderful to look forward to on a daily basis. Pre-cancer, I, like many others, did not make enough time for special times with loved ones as often as I should have. Surviving cancer has changed that, and now that time seems as important to me as the air I breathe and the water I drink. I only hope and pray I can give as much to each of them in return!

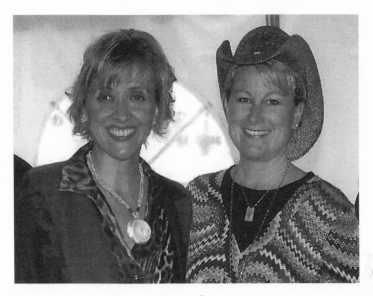

Laura and Lori
With My Wellness Partner Laura

In 2002, I wrote this poem for my loving "Wellness Partner" Connie while I was away in Africa. I re-dedicated these words to her, my dear Laura, and all those who walk with me on my journey...

For My Forever Friend

When I was looking for answers,
I found her.
When I need to see a smiling face,
hear words of encouragement and hope,
she is there.
She's taught me everything she knows
and embraces me with open arms;
we share a spirit only few others
could really understand.
She guides me along the way
with calmness and character;
bursting full of energy, love,
compassion and dignity.
Always putting others first,
never uttering an angry word;
with a genuine kindness others only aspire to.
Like the big sister I have never had,
she takes my hand and offers shelter under her wing;
with a desire to protect me,
to ensure my safety.
With the face of an angel,
she calms my fears;
her touch gives me strength…
together, we will win!

We both understand what life is about,

how precious it is;

how thankful we are for it.

We regard each day as a special gift,

and love with every ounce of our being.

Although we're terrified inside,

we try so hard to keep it in;

we want to be tough.

We laugh together,

we cry together;

and we are strong together.

First and foremost devoted wives,

loving mothers, special daughters and sisters but —

ALWAYS, FOREVER FRIENDS!

Chapter 11

The Power of the
Touched By Cancer Foundation

"October, 2001. I woke up this morning with so many ideas —ideas that turned into plans that will help so many others better understand cancer and what they can do about it."

Inspiration. I had an idea... I wanted to build a new home and donate our profit from the home to breast cancer research and awareness. Our subcontractors and suppliers had been asking us for over a year what they could do for John and me. Besides continuing with their prayers, this was the answer: we can use our own knowledge and resources to build a house to raise money for cancer causes! Of course the first person I approached to discuss my idea, was John. I believe he saw a spark in my eyes for the first time in eighteen months.

I had just become truly confident that I was not going to die, and I needed to follow through with my promises to God: each time I was scanned or x-rayed, I asked God to, "please spare me; please let me live and in return I promise to do everything I can to help others with their fight." This was the answer and the vehicle with which to follow through with my promises!

John seemed interested in the idea. I think he thought having this new "baby" in my life would also help to relieve the sadness I felt for not being able to have the child we were hoping to have together (due to the chemotherapy). The Building Awareness Designer Show Home would, in fact, be my "baby" to nurture.

My friends embraced the idea and they started falling into place to form the committees. Although many people told me I was crazy to ask her, Katie Harman, while still in her reign as Miss America 2002, agreed to attend the ribbon-cutting ceremony and also convey our message of hope on the national level! This was important, not only to me that someone of such prominence would be interested in getting involved with my brand new idea, but also because Katie's major platform and campaign as Miss America was to spread the message about the meaning of a "metastatic breast cancer" diagnosis. I had been trying to teach everyone I knew since April of 2000 what it meant to have metastatic breast cancer, so it was very significant that Katie Harman was already spreading this message on a national scale!

Together, John and I sought the help of many other dedicated individuals to assist us in getting things organized, so many more than I can name in one book. Many people desire to "give back" in any way they can; someone just needs to guide them along! At this point, God was clearly guiding me because this little "baby" was quickly growing into much more responsibility than I could ever handle on my own!

The Foundation. I was first advised by a childhood friend to start a 501(c) (3) foundation. I had never even heard of something like that before, unless it had to do with selling or building new homes, I felt like an idiot! However, as I did more research about the subject, I realized that the home would serve as the "foundation" (no pun intended!) of the not-for-profit foundation. The Building Awareness Designer Show Home's purpose was two-fold. First, the net proceeds from its sale would be the major source of funds for the Foundation and its work. Second it would serve as the vehicle in which to convey my messages of hope and education to others newly diagnosed.

Beyond knowing that the Show Home could provide the ways to a means, I knew little else about how to make things happen the "right" way. In order to accomplish the feats that lay ahead legally, morally and purposefully, I knew I would need help.

That's when God sent me another angel to help with the task. I knew when I met Brian Johnston, a Kansas City attorney, there was an immediate connection. We had both been "touched by cancer" way too many times and he was spiritually searching for a way to give back in memory of loved ones who had lost their fight to cancer. Brian took the lead, set up our foundation with the state, created our by-laws, and filed the necessary paperwork with the Internal Revenue Service to start the process in getting our "501(c)(3)" status. *(As a footnote to anyone that thinks of starting a foundation and believes that getting the necessary IRS approval is easy, it isn't: it is a very time-intensive process that takes several months to get approved and requires the help of people that know what they are doing to get it done right).* Brian not only got us started, but also continues today serving as an advisor to the Board of Directors.

I cannot stress how important it is for each new foundation to have a "Brian". I know I would have thrown my hands up many times since the beginning if not for his energy, drive and commitment to the foundation. Brian told me in the very beginning how much work it would be to run a non-profit foundation that relies solely upon the efforts and energies of volunteers to accomplish its purposes. I never dreamed it would be so much work! There are constant pressures to do your very best in raising funds to support your organization's purposes and causes, and you have to do so in a manner that is allowable by approved IRS guidelines. In addition, there are constant struggles to make sure there are enough volunteers to support the foundation's efforts, while at the same time not too heavily taxing the relationships of friends and family to make things happen. Brian and many others have always been there to help me keep our ultimate priorities straight. They have helped to spread the messages of hope and healing that we know are helping save lives for tomorrow that could not be saved yesterday based on the lack of knowledge of cancer treatment options and alternatives.

The Mission. The Touched by Cancer Foundation was created on January 24, 2002 (we originally organized as the Lori C. Lober Cancer Foundation, but later changed the name because we soon realized how many people have been "touched by cancer" in their lives, through themselves, a loved one or close family member or friend). The Foundation's mission was to become a comprehensive resource increasing cancer awareness and promoting positive treatment outcomes. We sought to accomplish this by:

- Educating newly diagnosed cancer patients about multiple opinions and correct diagnosis before treatment begins (it is particularly important to not pursue surgical removal or other surgical options until you know this is the absolute best alternative available);
- Creating awareness of National Cancer Institute designated Comprehensive Cancer Centers;
- Providing information to the community regarding all treatment options;
- Promoting overall health and wellness to those diagnosed with cancer or any other "at risk" individuals.

We continue to make strides forward in accomplishing our ultimate goal of ensuring that anyone diagnosed with cancer is fully equipped with the information they need to fight and win their battle against cancer. We have had very dedicated Board members (again, too many to name but we wouldn't be where we are without our past and present board members). While much has been accomplished, we are far from the finish line! Our current board and Wellness Center staff continue their efforts to fulfill our mission.

Building Awareness. The first-ever "BUILDING FOR A CURE DESIGNER SHOW HOME" built by Provence Homes, Inc. by John Lober, was completed in October, 2002. Local Kansas City businesses and interior designers decorated the home to provide a unique "show home" décor that encouraged the attendance of many who knew nothing about our foundation or its cancer-related purposes. Many subcontractors and suppliers to the home donated their time and products for the home so that the net profits from the sale of the home provided even more funds to support the Touched By Cancer Foundation's mission. The "Show Home" helped build awareness and funds by serving as a venue for several cancer-related events during Breast Cancer Awareness Month. Proceeds from the sale of that first home benefitted the University of Kansas School of Medicine Flaxseed Study (as an alternative to traditional chemotherapy approaches in breast cancer patients) by Dr. Carol Fabian and the University of Missouri at Kansas City's School of Medicine's establishment of a new comprehensive alternative medical center.

The second show home was also built by Provence Homes, Inc. by John Lober and was now referred to as the "Building Awareness Designer Show Home." The 2004 home presented a consistent decoration style and theme. The cancer battles of several prominent cancer survivors and celebrities were highlighted throughout the home. Additional information was made available that outlined each person's cancer and the available treatment options. Due to the popularity of the home and its events, the 2004 Show Home was sold within three weeks of its first public event! The proceeds from the 2004 Show Home have now supported additional contributions to other worthy causes, including M.D. Anderson's House of Wellness as well as Turning Point of Kansas City, the Center for Hope and Healing.

In the fulfillment of our mission, we've now built six homes. The third Building Awareness Designer Show Home opened to the public in August of 2005. The significance of the 2005 Show Home was not only its importance in raising funds, and in spreading the foundation's educational campaign and message to a new audience, but also because it was the first home that was built without the help and assistance of John or myself. A prominent Kansas City homebuilder, Tom French Construction, Inc., built the 2005 show home. The next two years saw the completion of two more Building Awareness Designer Show Homes. These homes were built by Brett and Corey Childress and Don Julian Builders, respectfully. The award winning 2008 Building Awareness Designer Show Home was completed by Lambie-Geer Homes.

Following the example of the preceding years, each home has showcased the unique talents and skill of our local building and design community. The homebuilder and the designers dedicated their work to individuals who have been touched by cancer. Visitors were invited to view these outstanding homes (which over the years have garnered much local and national publicity and many local awards for design and purpose), and were given valuable information about cancer and available treatment options. In particular, the foundation supplied an informative publication that conveyed useful information regarding breast cancer and the importance of early diagnosis.

There are not enough words to thank all of the people involved in bringing the Show Homes to completion. Our local communities of builders, artisans, designers, and volunteers have been and continue to be more than generous in supporting our mission to build cancer awareness and promote positive outcomes!

My personal dream is to take our "Show Home' concept outside of the Kansas City area, to spread our message of awareness, hope and healing throughout America. It is our goal that homebuilders across the country will continue to embrace our ideas and concepts to initiate similar events each and every year until cancer is torn down and demolished from our existence.

Moving Forward. After losing Colby so much shifted in my life. As the weeks and months passed, I had many dreams and inspirations come to me about how I could honor Colby's compassion, generosity, honesty and zest for life. One idea that came to me was to honor a young person who was dedicated to helping others just as Colby had chosen to do. My dear friend Laura urged me to listen to the inspiration and follow it. I approached the Director at Touched By Cancer about the idea of a scholarship fund and through the process emerged the Colby James McLain Memorial Scholarship Award. Now the Touched by Cancer Foundation awards a student volunteer who has contributed not only to the Foundation, but also to the broader community and our world with an annual scholarship in memory of Colby James McLain. Colby was our first volunteer and unconditionally supported my vision for the Touched By Cancer Foundation. His love, compassion and zest for life were evident to all who knew him. Colby touched many lives before his death in November, 2005. He'll continue to do so, in part through this award given in his honor.

Like any mission, ours requires lots of hands doing anything from answering telephones at the Foundation office, to event planning, to serving beverages at the Show Home ribbon cutting. Volunteers are an integral part of any non-profit foundation. Without the many dedicated hours given selflessly by volunteers in support of a common mission, much important work would be left undone. In honor of my brave brother Lance, The Lance C. Wittmeyer Memorial Award is presented annually to acknowledge the outstanding efforts of an individual who has made a difference in the lives of those who have been touched by cancer. Although Lance lost his battle with cancer, his courage inspired me to become actively engaged in my own diagnosis and treatment and to raise awareness of cancer while paying tribute to him.

On October 1, 2006, I officially moved to the Advisory Committee of the Touched By Cancer Foundation. After founding the organization and living it all day, every day for over four years I understood at this crucial time in my personal journey I needed to focus on my own health and well-being. The loss, hurt, emptiness and pain I felt even a year after losing Colby would make it very easy for me to crawl under the covers and give up. I did not want to do that. I wanted to keep the promises I have made since the beginning of my cancer journey.

I want to continue helping everyone I can who hears the dreaded words "you have cancer". Letting go of the hands-on responsibilities at the Foundation has enabled me to get together one-on-one with as many of those who need help while being true to my own journey. While I am doing well, I cannot afford to compromise my own wellness by staying too busy to take care of myself. After all, I should practice what I preach!

A Dream Come True. After the first publication of **Bigger Than Pink**, both the foundation and I received multiple phone inquiries from cancer patients and their caregivers. They wanted to know how to integrate complementary therapies into a wellness plan, how to find the right practitioners and how to talk to Western physicians about complementary therapies.

After hearing about these phone calls the Board of Directors began working on a solution to help people with cancer and their caregivers find affordable complementary therapies. It became obvious to the Board of Directors that the most logical solution would be to provide these services at a new Touched By Cancer Wellness Center. In early 2007, the Touched By Cancer Foundation launched a pilot program at our new Wellness Center. Complementary therapies were offered at a highly subsidized rate to cancer patients as well as a full slate of free educational classes open to anyone touched by cancer. The pilot program confirmed that there was a demand for complementary therapies, a desire for education about how to incorporate them into a cancer journey, and a need for subsidized rates. We also found that many practitioners were looking for an outlet to help those really in need. The pilot program offered those on a cancer journey an affordable outlet to learn about and try complementary therapies.

With the success of the pilot program, the Touched By Cancer Foundation has adjusted its focus to provide more direct programming to people with cancer and their caregivers. Our mission has expanded to:

> *"The Touched By Cancer Foundation is a source of inspiration, information and wellness for those whose lives have been touched by cancer."*

Our programming has expanded and become more defined. Currently, the Touched By Cancer Foundation offers:

- **Educational Programming-** Nutrition, Introduction to Complementary Modalities, Meditation, Sharing Our Stories, Stress Reduction, Literature Review, etc.

- **Informative Events and Resources-** Wellness a la Carte (a sampling of complementary modalities), and upgrades to the Touched By Cancer Foundation website allowing clients of the Touched By Cancer Foundation to schedule appointments, participate in community message boards and create their own cancer information packets. Any web user has access to the website's services and information.
- **Complementary Therapies-** Therapeutic Massage, Acupressure, Acupuncture, Comfort Touch Therapy, Wellness Counseling, Reflexology, Chiropractic Services, Guided Imagery and Energy Healing.

The number of patients and caregivers receiving services from the Touched By Cancer Foundation has increased at a sustainable growth rate of 20% throughout 2008. At the time of this writing, the Touched By Cancer Foundation is exploring partnerships with other agencies serving those touched by cancer and has been approached by some local hospitals to provide educational programming and potentially complementary therapies on site. In addition, the Foundation sponsors other fund-raising events in Kansas City and participates with other local organizations' cancer and health and wellness-related educational events.

Yes, the Touched by Cancer Foundation has truly been a "labor" of love and has ultimately helped me focus on helping others. It truly helps me fulfill my purpose and brings meaning to my life. It is my vehicle to touch other lives and "give back". Each time I tell my story I am encouraged to stay on my long-term path to wellness. It's not just about going through the motions; having surgery, having chemotherapy, being tested, going to doctors' appointments, day in and day out. There is so much more to it. Eating correctly, continuing on my journey of overall optimal health and wellness, living each day to the fullest, enjoying my friends and family like I never did "before cancer" is what I am about now and what I intend to be about for many, many years to come!

Chapter 12

The Power of Being Happy, Being Healthy, Loving and Being Loved!

He formed a triangle with his hands and said, "...Each of the three sides of the triangle are equal – when they're all equal and they meet, that's when we experience the best life has to offer."

Colby James McLain

Just prior to the first release of **Bigger Than Pink** in early 2006, I lost Colby, my only child in an early morning car accident. I was told he hit a piece of black ice and his car hit a tree head-on. I was assured by so many that Colby never felt any pain.

But – for me – I wondered why?? Why, after living through a stage four, metastatic breast cancer diagnosis was I left here, while my brilliant, thriving, loving and beautiful son is gone? I had two choices. I could choose to live my life to the fullest or I could sink into a deep, dark hole of depression. My husband and dearest, best friends (you know who you are) have witnessed my moments of grieving – often times surfacing when I least expected it. I believe Colby is safe and sound in Heaven and he guides me and gives me strength every day.

Colby was born November 21, 1986. His birthday always fell right before Thanksgiving. He was home with us celebrating the Thanksgiving holiday. I will always remember him walking in for his last Thanksgiving dinner, dressed in nicely pressed jeans and a crisp, white, button-down collared shirt. I was so proud of my son who wanted so badly to be medical doctor who also truly understood how well Eastern modalities could complement the best Western medicine has to offer.

He had cut off all his curls on his 19th birthday. He looked like he had matured in so many ways since moving into the dorm at University of Missouri Kansas City. I was so proud that he, on his own, had decided to make this transformation. He was very well known for his big, curly locks!

After our meal, Colby asked if we would mind that he and Anthony, John's eldest son, went down to the Country Club Plaza to witness the annual Christmas lighting ceremony. Since Colby was very young he had been drawn to the Plaza! We were fine with it. They went, met some of Colby's college friends from UMKC and came straight back home. Colby never wanted to miss the family playing Balderdash together and that is just what we did that night! He always won! I was amazed and stunned at his wittiness and creativity!

The next day, Colby asked permission to have some of his high school buddies over, to hang out and spend the night. I was honored they all came and had wonderful conversations reminiscing about the "old days" now that they were all college students! John and I went to bed and fell soundly asleep knowing all of Colby's friends were spending the night. Something awoke me and I wandered half asleep into the hallway where I caught a glimpse of Colby's naked back. He had swimming trunks on because they had been in the hot tub.

I gasped when I saw a tattoo on his upper back. Basically, a triangle with angel wings. This caught me totally off guard as we had discussed tattoos previously and he knew I was opposed to him having one. How would that look if anyone ever knew their doctor had a tattoo? Colby calmed me down and we decided he and I would discuss it Saturday morning after his friends left.

I will never forget this conversation until the day I see Colby in Heaven. Colby explained to me that he had always regarded life as a triangle, not a circle. He formed a triangle with his two hands and said,

"Mom, you more than anyone will understand this! Each of the three sides of the triangle is equal – when they're all equal and they meet, that's when we experience the best life has to offer."

"Each of these sides," his hands forming a triangle as he revealed his mantra, "this side is Being Happy, this side is Being Healthy, and this side is Loving and Being Loved. Mom, that's how I live my life!"

I'll have to admit at that moment I was speechless. My son had just taught me something that would sustain my belief in faith and hope for the rest of MY life!

So, my next question was, "Well, what's the deal with the angel wings?"

He didn't waste a second. He said, "Mom, those are to carry me to Heaven, whenever that may be."

Again, I was so caught off guard I didn't have a very good comeback. Bottom line, my son was an amazing spirit that will live on forever. Many of my friends also believe he helps guide them on a regular basis. (I celebrated Colby's memory by tattooing his name on the inside of my left ankle on the 20th anniversary of Colby's birth and love it! He would too!)

I strive to live the best life I can, based on Colby's triangle mantra! For me, cancer has been a big fork in the road, dealing with the loss of my only, beautiful child has been a journey I would never wish on another human being. When I feel stress or witness others feeling stress, I know it sounds crazy, but I think to myself, "I am so glad my son experiences no stress." As a parent, we don't want our children to hurt and in my heart I know that Colby can never be hurt.

Colby and Mackenzie Crosby had been dating for 2 ½ years before we lost Colby. John and I met Kenzie when she had just turned 15. Colby and Kenzie were truly our first Touched By Cancer Foundation volunteers and even attended the Touched By Cancer Foundation events and galas with us! John and I were just positive Kenzie would, after college, be our daughter-in-law. We feel blessed every day to know Kenzie will forever be our "Daughter-In- Love!"

After losing Colby, I could not stand the thought of Kenzie pulling away and losing her too. After all, John and I have been able to witness her mature into a beautiful, loving, giving and thriving young woman! Kenzie and Colby's best childhood friend, Matt, joined us on our annual family vacation the spring of 2006 after losing Colby. That trip was hard for us and at the same time, healing for us. Even now, we still break down at times. Most importantly, we remember Colby's zest for life and try to live the way he would want us to. We celebrated 07-07-07 in his honor and just recently 08-08-08. As crazy as it sounds, his favorite jersey numbers were 7 and 8! I know he was smiling down from Heaven on those glorious nights!

Colby had been my rock, my strength, my soul-mate for 19 years and 1 week. I admired him for his wit, his intelligence, his work ethic, his ability to make everyone he knew feel loved and valued. He was kind, at times even too generous, musically gifted and he lit up every room he entered with his smile, his warmth and his honesty. He gave the BEST hugs! So, yes, losing Colby impacts every day of my life. And, I have made a conscious decision to "Be Happy, Be Healthy, To Love and Be Loved" until I see my sweet Angel in Heaven! I invite you to do the same!

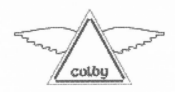

Conclusion

On January 2, 2009, I saw my oncologist for my annual scans. While I am confident in my wellness and feel better that I have ever felt, I cannot help but be a bit nervous each time the tests are run. Since I was leaving for a trip the next day, my oncologist assured me he would do everything he could to get the scans read and call me with the results before I left. After my appointment, I joined my editor to review photographs and the final draft of **Still Bigger Than Pink**. As our meeting came to a close, my cell phone rang… it was a call from my oncologist's office. They had *great* news, all was clear and there continues to be no evidence of disease! The spot on my hip they have been watching has even shrunk in the last year! I know dedication to self-care and my new IsAgenix regimen are working to create balance in my body allowing for optimum healing!

My doctors cannot give me definite answers as to why my treatments have been successful when others have failed, or even why I'm still alive and thriving. However, they have said many times that I "am a very proactive patient." Of course, being proactive does not guarantee success and long-term survival – unfortunately, there are no guarantees. However, I feel that truly believing that I was not going to die, most certainly was an important factor. In addition to that, my faith, the support of my family and friends, the combination of everything discussed in this book, and yes, a little luck, have all contributed to my long-term survival. Prior to being diagnosed with cancer, I would not necessarily have considered myself an extraordinarily lucky person. Now the quality of life I live every day is much richer, the special moments more memorable, and the love I have to offer both to myself as well as to others, is deeper and more fulfilling. This is precisely why I tell everyone I meet that I feel "blessed" to have actually had cancer, and I continue to be deeply grateful to now be healthy and happy.

Journey well!

xoxo,
Lori

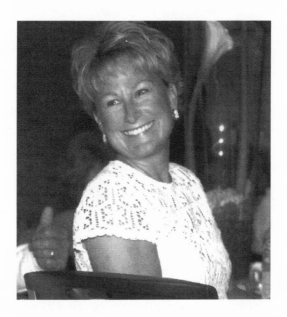

My Journey

11/29/95

First Mammogram – "Dense breasts with micro calcifications - no cancer".

1998

Second mammogram – 11/20/98 – "negative for cancer" Appointment with OB/GYN – one suspicious area
Appointment with first surgeon – would need a biopsy to "rule out" cancer – thought the suspicious area was "probably not cancer". Sought second opinion.
Two appointments with second surgeon – No need for biopsy it was "fibrous dysplasia; nothing to worry about."

April 10, 2000

Third Mammogram – Negative for cancer – I felt something was not right.

April 13, 2000

First appointment with third surgeon – First biopsy – indicated I had "Ductal Carcinoma in situ".

April 20, 2000

Second appointment with third surgeon – Second biopsy (To rule out Inflammatory Breast Cancer).

April 24, 2000
First appointment with Oncologist at M.D. Anderson Cancer Center in Houston, Texas.

April 24-28, 2000
Ongoing testing to determine "stage". 7 cm. x 4 cm. breast tumor confirmed. Positive "nodes" revealed during fine needle aspiration. Inflammatory breast cancer ruled out via core biopsies. CT scan positive for liver metastasis. Meetings with breast multi-disciplinary team of doctors at MDACC.

April 28, 2000
Diagnosis of Stage IV breast cancer with metastasis (spread) to the liver
– THE WORST DAY OF MY LIFE, at that point.

May 1, 2000
Surgical insertion of first catheter and first chemotherapy treatment at MDACC – Taxotere/Herceptin Clinical Trial paperwork signed.

May, 2000
My brother, Lance, passes away of cancer. I fight to live in honor of him. Had it not been for Lance, I would not know that comprehensive cancer centers exist; something I wish we had learned years earlier to aid him in his fight.

June, July, August, 2000
Taxotere/Herceptin Chemotherapy continues.

September 28, 2000
Liver surgery at MDACC – experimental Radio Frequency Ablation – Believed by my multi-disciplinary team to be successful!

October, 2000
More chemotherapy – Herceptin/Taxotere.

November 10, 2000
Double mastectomy – MDACC – no reconstruction.

Thanksgiving, 2000
On vacation with my mother and Colby in Cabo San Lucas recuperating from the two surgeries. (I believe "getting away from it all" can be very healing!)

December, 2000
More chemotherapy – Herceptin/Taxotere.

January 1, 2001
"DATELINE" special featuring "metastatic breast cancer guru" Dr. Yeshi Dhonden.

January, February, March, 2001
Adriamyacin, Cytoxin, 5-FU Regime.

Summer/Fall, 2001
Navelbene Experimental Chemotherapy Regime – (I was scared to quit!).

Spring, 2002
DUKE Immunization Study in North Carolina – involved 6 trips to Durham, NC. What an honor to participate in yet another clinical trial!

Summer, 2002
Double-doses of Herceptin every 21 days begin.

2002-2009
Herceptin continues. Reflexology treatments, therapeutic massage, colonics, acupuncture, chiropractic alignment, proper nutrition, herbal supplementation and Tibetan herbs continue. Appointments with Dr. Yeshi Dhonden annually or as he is available; re-evaluation and follow-up.

Although PET scans show a "hot spot" at my left hip area, I continue to thrive. I am medically diagnosed as "no evidence of disease".

2003
Honored as a *Yoplait Champion* in the fight against cancer by SELF Magazine and the Susan G. Komen Foundation.

2004
Honored as an *Outstanding Missourian* – What a privilege!

2005
Spelman campaign for digital mammography equipment
April, Colby accepted into med school
Spring, Began advocating for clinical trials for the Biotechnology industry.
November 28 Losing Colby – *The Worst Day of My Life.*

2007
Became "Her Story" Ambassador for Genentech
May, guest @ Biotech Convention
September, special guest at Kansas City Life Science Event

January 2, 2009, Still no evidence of disease! AND the hot spot on my hip is finally smaller!

April 30, 2009, I was honored to speak at Duke. I remain overwhelmed with their dedication and support of me and my cancer journey. This is truly a world-class institution in every way!

I continue with on-going bone scans, PET scans, x-rays, echo-cardiogram studies, etc. as needed and ordered by my oncologist. I strive to eliminate daily stress (the main thing doctors say can cause the metastasis to flare quickly and aggressively return) with regular body work, proper nutrition and living Colby's mantra...

"Be Happy, Be Healthy, To Love and Be Loved!"

Resources

Cancer Information:

National Cancer Institute (NCI)
NCI Public Inquiries Office
6116 Executive Boulevard, Room 3036A
Bethesda, MD 20892-8322
1-800-4-CANCER
www.cancer.gov

Oncolink Editorial Board
Abramson Cancer Center of the University of Pennsylvania
3400 Spruce Street – 2 Donner
Philadelphia, PA 19104-4283
Fax: 215-349-5445
www.oncolink.org

American Cancer Society
1-800-ACS-2345
www.cancer.org

Touched By Cancer Foundation
4770 N. Belleview Avenue, Suite 201
Kansas City, MO 64116
Phone: 816-505-0040
Fax: 816-505-7264
www.touchedbycancerfoundation.org

Complementary and Holistic Medicine:

National Institutes of Health
National Center for Complementary and Alternative Medicine
6707 Democracy Boulevard, Suite 401
Bethesda, MD 20892-5475
(888) 644-6226
www.nccam.nih.gov

Duke Integrative Medicine
3475 Erwin Road
Durham, NC 27710
919-660-6827
www.dukeintegrativemedicine.org

American Holistic Health Association
P.O. Box 17400
Anaheim, CA 92817
714-779-6152
www.ahha.org

American Holistic Medical Association
6728 Old McLean Village Drive
McLean, VA 22101
703-556-9728
www.holisticmedicine.org

International Chiropractic Association
1110 N. Glebe Rd
Suite 650
Arlington, VA 22201
800-423-4690
www.chiropractic.org

Acupuncture:

American Academy of Medical Acupuncture
5820 Wilshire Boulevard
Los Angeles, CA 90036
213-937-5514
www.medicalacupuncture.org

American Association of Oriental Medicine
433 Front Street
Catasqua, PA 18032
610-266-1433
www.aaom.org

Reflexology :

International Institute of Reflexology
P.O. Box 12462
St. Petersburg, FL 33733
813-343-4811
www.reflexology-usa.net

Therapeutic Touch:

Nurse Healers Professional Associates
1211 Locust Street
Philadelphia, PA 19107
215-545-8079
www.therapeutic-touch.org

Colon Therapy:

International Association for Colon Hydrotherapy
P.O. Box 461285
San Antonio, TX 78246
210-366-2888
www.i-act.org

Nutritional and Cellular Cleansing:

IsAgenix
www.johnlober.isagenix.com

Dr. Tony O'Donnell, N.D.
www.radiantgreens.com
888.456.1597
Email: doctony@radiantgreens.com

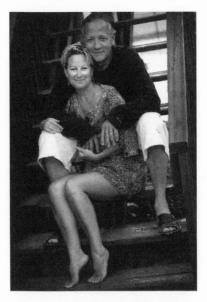

(Photo by Tracy Routh Photography)

About the Author

Lori Lober's personal brush with cancer came in 1998, when she found a suspicious lump in her breast. A doctor's visit revealed that the lump was a non-cancerous fibrocystic disease. In 2000, after feeling increasingly ill since her examinations beginning two years earlier, Lori went to yet another doctor. By this time, she was finally diagnosed as a stage four breast cancer patient and the disease had metastasized to her liver. Lori was given 12 to 18 months to live.

Traditional cancer treatments at that time offered little hope of long-term survival. The odds she would even be alive five years later were less than 3 percent. Lori was determined to beat the odds. She conducted extensive research and created an integrative treatment plan incorporating the best of Western conventional medicine with complementary therapies. This research also led her to a Comprehensive Cancer Center with an innovative team of doctors and a clinical trial that included a biological therapy that attacked her cancer cells while leaving her healthy cells unharmed.

Her tumors responded well to the treatment and nine years later there is no evidence of the disease in her body.

The life-altering experience left Lori deeply touched by the support she received from her husband, friends and family, inspiring her to form the Touched by Cancer Foundation to help and give hope to others "touched by cancer". Her first book, *Bigger Than Pink: The Book I Could Not Find When I Was Diagnosed With Stage IV Cancer*, includes her personal journey of combining both Eastern and Western medicine. Lori continues to thrive and has been an active advocate for integrative care, biotechnology, clinical trials and optimal health and wellness through nutrition.

Lori is happily married to her Prince Charming, John Lober. Both passionate animal lovers and activists, together they enjoy traveling and spending time with family and friends. John and Lori Lober live in Kansas City, Missouri.

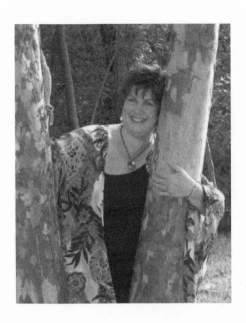

About Teresa Kelly

Teresa's cancer journey began in 2006. Soon after surgery she received *Bigger Than Pink* by Lori Lober. Having assembled a wellness plan that included conventional and complementary therapies, she found Lori's book affirming and inspirational. She met Lori later that year and eventually became a volunteer for the Touched By Cancer Foundation. Furthering her commitment to the principles that kept her healthy during treatment, Teresa continues to advocate for the development of integrative treatment plans that empower those on a wellness journey.

Her company, Good Natured Living, assists others in their quest to live consciously in balance with the planet. She promotes wellness, a sustainable lifestyle and environmental awareness through her writing, organic gardening, cooking experiences, and retreats/workshops.

Teresa is married to the man of her dreams and mother to four wonderful children. Through her own cancer journey, Teresa has learned to live life fully in each moment.

Made in the USA
Middletown, DE
14 November 2014